HEALTHY GUT
DIET GUIDE
+COOKBOOK

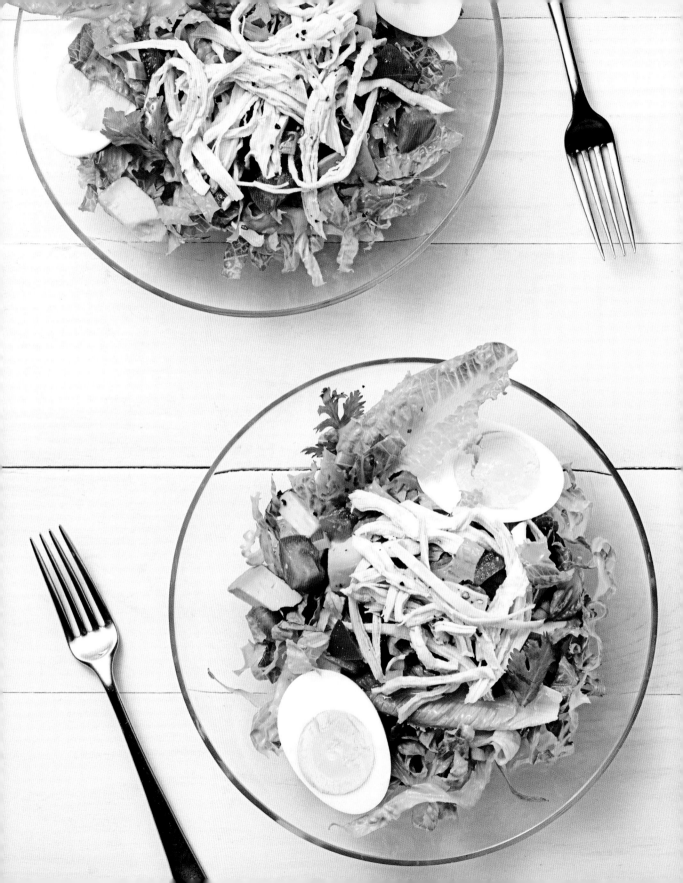

More Than 175 Healing Recipes
to Improve Your Digestive Health

HEALTHY GUT
DIET GUIDE
+COOKBOOK

Maya Gangadharan, FNTP

Contents

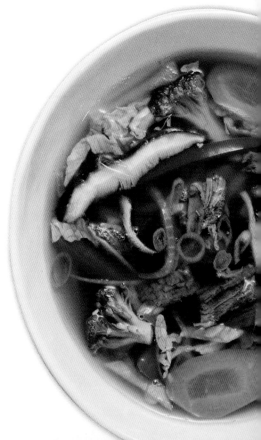

Introduction

We've all heard phrases referencing the relationship between your innards and your emotions, such as "gut feeling." Recently, medical professionals have begun to explore the connection between your gut and your health.

Leaky Gut Syndrome

Recent studies have linked the microbiome—another word for the world of friendly (and sometimes unfriendly) bacteria and microbes that live in your intestines—to weight loss, depression, Alzheimer's disease, autism, and more. Problems like gas, bloating, constipation, and diarrhea often are thought of as normal, but in fact, they often are symptoms of a "leaky gut" that has become compromised by stress, bad habits, bad food choices, or toxins. It's best to correct the problem before deeper issues develop.

The GAPS Diet

This book focuses on a gut-healing protocol called the Gut and Psychology Syndrome™, or GAPS, diet. The GAPS diet was created to address specific physical and physiological gut-related health issues. This book was written and designed to make that somewhat complicated protocol easier to understand and implement, and to give you more recipe options.

Based on the Specific Carbohydrate Diet (SCD), the GAPS diet was developed by neurologist and nutritionist Dr. Natasha Campbell-McBride. Her book, *Gut and Psychology Syndrome,* outlines the science of the protocol, and you're encouraged to read it to understand in detail how the gut becomes unbalanced and why the diet works. You also can visit gapsdiet.com for more information. There, you can find a certified GAPS practitioner if you decide you want a bit more guidance.

Other Related Diets

Several other diets share similarities with the GAPS diet and are used to treat health issues that stem from the gut. Like GAPS, the *Paleo diet* focuses on reducing carbohydrates, avoiding grains and refined sugar, and increasing nutrient-dense whole foods. One of the ways it differs from GAPS is that it does not allow dairy products. The *low-FODMAP diet* is another protocol for gut healing that focuses on eliminating particular carbohydrates, such as certain sugars. One way it differs from GAPS is in the list of allowed foods. Because you might be incorporating elements of other diets into your protocols, icons are included on this book's recipes to denote whether they are compatible with the Paleo or low-FODMAP diets.

The Basics of Healing

This book begins with an overview of how digestion is supposed to work and what can go wrong. We then review the basics of both the healing process and the diet itself, as well as offer advice on how to prepare your kitchen and pantry for a healthy gut. From there, we walk through each stage of the introduction diet, from stage 1 to stage 6, and explain how to transition to the full GAPS diet. Don't skip over this part; you'll want to be familiar with each stage and what you can expect before you begin.

ICONS

Throughout the recipes, you'll see various icons. Here's what they mean:

 PEANUT- AND NUT-FREE RECIPE This icon denotes recipes that are free of peanuts and tree nuts.

NUT FREE

 DAIRY-FREE RECIPE This icon indicates recipes that do not call for animal-sourced dairy products.

DAIRY FREE

 PALEO-FRIENDLY RECIPE This icon indicates recipes that are suitable for those who also are following the Paleo diet.

PALEO DIET

 LOW-FODMAP RECIPE This icon denotes recipes that are acceptable for readers following the low-FODMAP diet.

LOW FODMAP

Allergies and Sensitivities

Leaky gut syndrome can cause allergic reactions and intolerances to particular food types. Not everyone has the same allergies and intolerances, so icons are included on recipes that are free of the two most commonly reacted-to food groups: nuts and dairy (or those ingredients are listed as optional). If you are unsure of your intolerances, instructions are provided for two common tests in the "Going Forward on the Diet" section. As your gut heals, you may be able to reintroduce dairy, and steps for doing that are provided in the same section.

The Path to Feeling Better

Most people notice positive results within the first couple stages. Those with deeper healing issues might have to wait a little longer or need subsequent rounds of the introduction diet to complete the healing process. Although the first few stages are restricted, the later stages and the full GAPS diet are full of delicious foods that taste great and help support vibrant health. Good luck on your journey!

Healing in Stages

The diet is very specific about what foods can be eaten when, so the recipes are organized by stage, indicated by icons. Be sure to follow the protocol strictly. Don't add foods earlier than they're allowed, or you risk compromising your healing. You always can go back to earlier recipes after you've moved on from that stage.

Stage 1 Focuses on stocks, boiled meats, some well-cooked vegetables, and cultured dairy.

Stage 4 Allows roasted and baked meats and fish, fresh juices, and some seed and nut flours.

Stage 2 Allows the addition of raw egg yolks, stews, herbs, and ghee.

Stage 5 Reintroduces apples, raw vegetables as in salads, fruit juice, and other spices and nut flours.

Stage 3 Allows you to add avocado, cooked eggs, asparagus, and a few other vegetables.

Stage 6 Allows more raw fruits, Brazil nuts, and more sweet baked goods.

Full diet This is the maintenance phase, which allows greater variety but continues to restrict some foods.

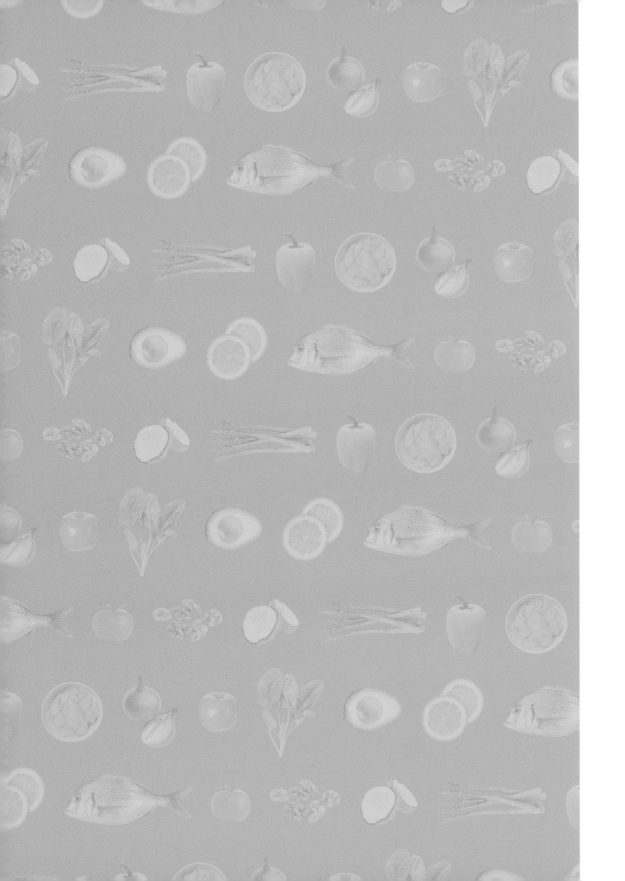

Understanding Gut Health

When things go wrong in your gut, it affects the rest of your body as well as your mind. In this part, you learn about leaky gut syndrome and how the right diet can put you on the path to healing.

When Digestion Goes Wrong

Leaky gut syndrome occurs when the lining of the small intestine becomes too permeable, causing a cascade of immune responses that can lead to chronic health problems. This permeability can be due to inflammatory foods such as gluten, dairy, sugar, and alcohol; some medications; intestinal parasites; and even stress.

1 Brain

- **NORMAL FUNCTION** Digestion actually begins in the brain, when you see, smell, or sometimes even think of food. Your mouth begins to water, and your body begins to prepare the various digestive organs to receive and process food.

- **WHAT CAN GO WRONG** This step of digestion can go wrong when you're eating under stress—in the car, during a meeting, or while doing chores—which puts your body in fight-or-flight rather than rest-and-digest mode and hampers the digestive process from the very beginning.

2 Mouth

- **NORMAL FUNCTION** In the mouth, food is broken down mechanically by chewing and chemically by enzymes present in saliva.

- **WHAT CAN GO WRONG** If you gulp down your food instead of chewing it properly, you force your stomach to do more work. That stresses your digestive system and can result in food being improperly digested.

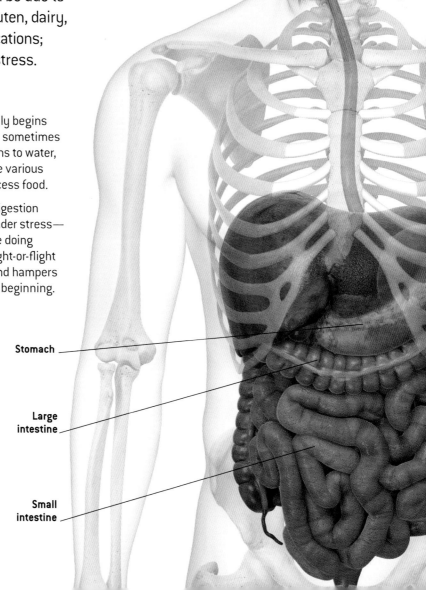

Brain

Mouth

Stomach

Large intestine

Small intestine

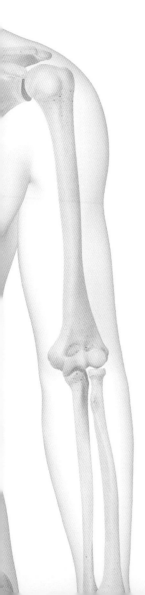

3 Stomach

- **NORMAL FUNCTION** Your stomach breaks down food mechanically by contracting the muscles of the stomach wall and chemically by using stomach acid and digestive enzymes.

- **WHAT CAN GO WRONG** It's very common for a person to underproduce (rather than overproduce, as commonly believed) stomach acid, which can lead to problems like heartburn and acid reflux and contribute to leaky gut and food allergies.

4 Small Intestine

- **NORMAL FUNCTION** The small intestine is where most of the digestion of nutrients takes place. The lining of the small intestine is designed to be permeable so properly digested food can be absorbed into the bloodstream and lymphatic system and circulated around the body.

- **WHAT CAN GO WRONG** Leaky gut occurs when the lining becomes too permeable, allowing undigested food particles, toxins, and microbes into the bloodstream, where the body attacks them as foreign invaders.

5 Large Intestine

- **NORMAL FUNCTION** A small amount of nutrient absorption occurs in the large intestine. In addition, the large intestine reabsorbs water from the food, and beneficial bacteria in the large intestine convert waste into nutrients before the food is expelled as feces.

- **WHAT CAN GO WRONG** If you're dehydrated, your large intestine will hold feces as your body tries to reabsorb as much water as possible, causing constipation. If there's not enough beneficial bacteria in the colon, opportunistic bacteria can overwhelm the environment, causing gut dysbiosis.

LEAKY GUT SYNDROME

Leaky gut is believed to cause many physical and physiological issues. Stress, diet, inflammation, candida, and zinc deficiencies are all considered possible causes.

HEALTHY GUT

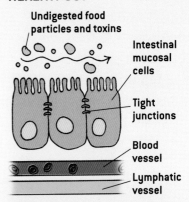

Healthy gut Junctions between mucosal cells lining the small intestine are tight and do not allow toxins to reach the bloodstream.

LEAKY GUT

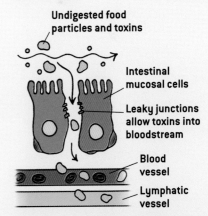

Leaky gut It is believed junctions become too permeable, allowing toxins to escape into the blood, causing a cascade of symptoms.

The Five R's of Gut Healing

When attempting to heal a leaky gut, it's best to go about things in a systematic way. By using a strategic protocol, you can ensure you cover all the bases on your way to good gut health. Functional medicine breaks the process down into the "five R's of gut healing." First, you **remove** foods that cause inflammation to the gut lining. Next, you systematically add back foods and supplements to **replace** digestive enzymes, **reinoculate** your gut with beneficial bacteria, and **repair** the damage with healing foods. Then you can **rebalance** your system with relaxing lifestyle changes.

Remove

ELIMINATE INFLAMMATORY FOODS FROM YOUR DIET

• Begin by removing foods that may be causing inflammation and damage to your gut. This includes certain foods that might trigger allergic reactions, such as grains, soy, eggs, and dairy, or foods that feed undesirable gut flora, such as sugar.

• Minimize exposure to environmental toxins such as smoke, household chemicals, and other pollutants.

• Reduce emotional stress. Yoga, meditation, and deep breathing all help promote a calm state of being.

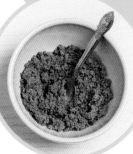

Sugars and other carbs contribute to an overgrowth of bad gut flora, so eliminating them is the first step.

Replace

ADD BACK ACIDS AND ENZYMES FOR BETTER DIGESTION

• Supplement with hydrochloric acid (HCl) to bolster low stomach acid production.

• Consider supplementing with digestive enzymes (available at health food stores) to aid digestion and help with assimilation of nutrients.

• Use digestive bitters (available at health food stores) to energize and tone your entire digestive system.

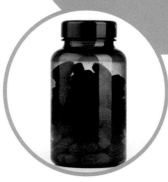

Supplements such as digestive enzymes can help your digestive system function better.

Reinoculate

SUPPLEMENT GOOD BACTERIA THROUGH PROBIOTICS

- You can add beneficial bacterial by taking a GAPS-friendly probiotic supplement.

- Eat probiotic foods, such as fermented vegetables, yogurt, and cultured cream.

- Drink probiotic beverages, such as kefir.

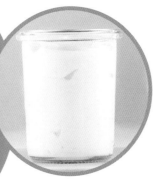

Homemade yogurt contains good bacteria that help balance your gut's microbiome.

Repair

FIX GUT DAMAGE WITH SUPPORTIVE FOODS

- Homemade stock and bone broths contain gelatin, which is soothing and helps repair the gut lining.

- Omega-3 fatty acids help reduce inflammation.

- In extreme cases, consult with a certified GAPS practitioner or other qualified medical professional for further supplementation.

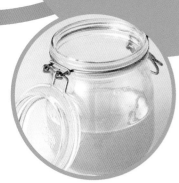

Homemade stock contains gelatin and fatty acids to repair leaky gut.

Rebalance

MAKE CALMING LIFESTYLE CHANGES

- When you eat, be sure you do so in a calm, relaxed state, which makes your digestive system more effective. Eat slowly, put down your fork between bites, and chew your food thoroughly.

- Consider incorporating yoga, meditation, breathwork, or other biofeedback practices to increase relaxation. Be sure to schedule time to unwind.

- Consider professional help if you're having trouble managing your stress level and emotional responses.

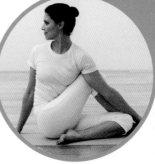

Yoga is one way to relax and calm your system so it functions better.

Pillars of the Diet

A core selection of healing foods supply the nutrients your gut needs. Some require special preparation ahead of time so they're ready to eat when you reach the later diet stages and you can tolerate them.

Healthy Fats

WHAT Lard, tallow, duck or chicken fat, responsibly and sustainably sourced coconut oil and palm oil, and ghee.

WHY Healthy fats are integral to gut healing. Although fats have been demonized for decades, research has started to catch up with the traditional viewpoint of fats as nutrient-dense, health-building foods.

HOW If you've been eating a low-fat diet, you may have difficulty digesting fats because your gallbladder and liver have become lazy at bile production. Start with a small amount, add beets to your diet to support the production of bile, and temporarily supplement with ox bile as your body adjusts.

Ghee is a healthy fat. Although it's made from dairy, it does not contain casein and lactose and is more tolerable for some.

Stocks and broths provide healing gelatin to repair intestinal damage.

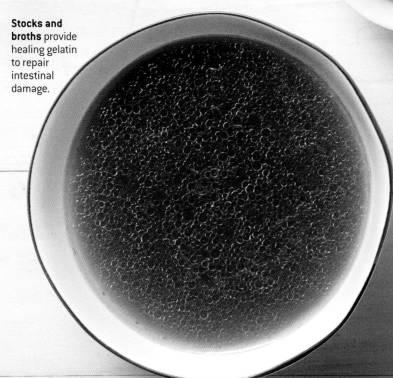

Stocks and Broths

WHAT Stocks and broths.

WHY Stock and its longer-cooking cousin, bone broth, are exceptionally healing to the gut lining. Gelatin, which comes from the collagen in bones, soothes inflammation and helps the gut repair more quickly. Stocks and broths also are excellent sources of amino acids and protein and help stretch your budget.

HOW Add meaty bones and stock to purified water. An acid, such as apple cider vinegar or lemon juice, helps bring out the minerals from the bones.

Meat

WHAT Meat, poultry, seafood, and animal fats.

WHY Animal products are incredibly dense in the vitamins and minerals your gut needs to heal properly.

HOW Choose grass-fed, pastured, or wild-caught animal products when possible. Animals are healthiest when they're eating the diet they were designed to eat, and the healthier the animal is, the healthier it will be for you. Always try to buy animal products free of extra hormones, which interfere with your endocrine system or cause allergic reactions.

Red meats are a diet staple, and provide key vitamins and minerals.

Fermented Vegetables

WHAT Sauerkraut, cultured vegetables, and pickles.

WHY Fermented foods are heavy hitters in the battle to heal your gut. The fermentation process allows beneficial bacteria to multiply, and eating the vegetables transfers the healthy microbes to your digestive tract. Fermentation also boosts the vegetables' vitamin and mineral content.

HOW You can ferment with just vegetables, salt, and filtered water, or you can add a starter culture. In the first few stages of the diet, you add the juice from cultured vegetables to soup. In later stages, as your gut heals enough to handle more fibrous foods, you consume the vegetables themselves. For long-term balance, plan on consuming fermented foods with every meal.

Cultured Dairy

WHAT Yogurt, kefir, cultured cream, cultured butter, and crème fraîche.

WHY Cultured dairy is another easy and delicious way to get beneficial probiotics into your gut. Many people who have trouble eating dairy can tolerate cultured dairy.

HOW To make cultured dairy, you need the appropriate starter culture, which you can find at health food stores or online. After you culture for the first time, you can use the finished product to start your next batch, making it very affordable. Use raw milk from an experienced farmer, or look for organic, grass-fed dairy that's been minimally pasteurized and homogenized.

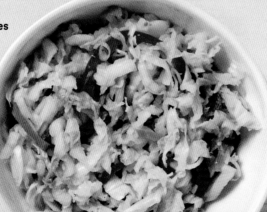

Cultured dairy such as yogurt adds back beneficial probiotics.

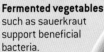

Fermented vegetables such as sauerkraut support beneficial bacteria.

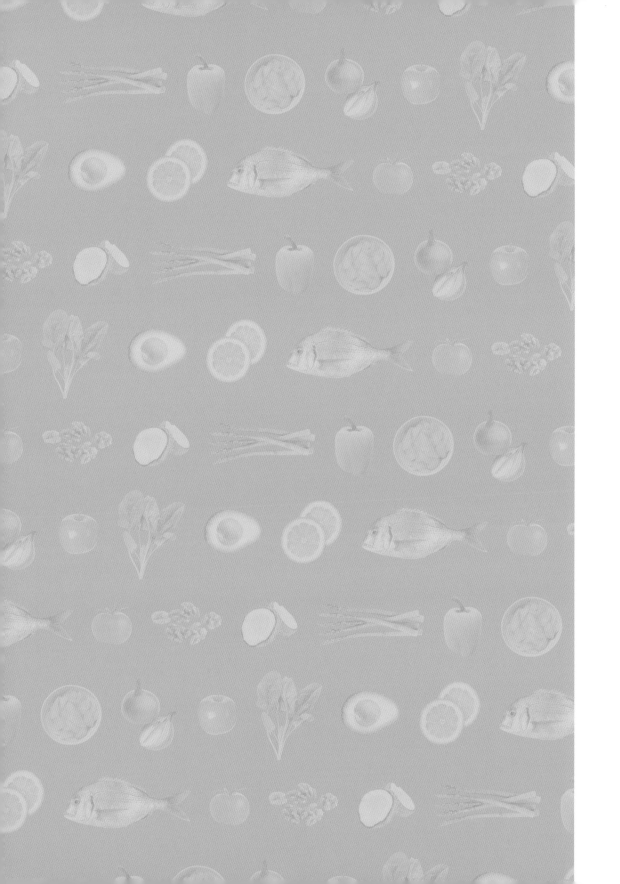

The Healthy Gut Diet

The GAPS diet is a specific protocol that begins with a six-stage introduction diet before you get to the full diet. In this part, you learn how to prepare for the diet and which foods are allowed at the various stages.

What to Expect

To reverse leaky gut and microbial imbalance (dysbiosis), you go through a healing crisis caused by "die-off," when the pathogenic bacteria start to die and leave your system. This is uncomfortable but normal.

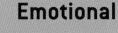

All Over

It's normal to be tired and feverish as your body works to repair itself. As you progress, you'll be amazed at the energy you feel as your body begins to digest and absorb nutrients more effectively.

Emotional

As your body rebalances, it can be overwhelming to cope with the symptoms of die-off and detoxification. Know where you can get support when you need it. For example, turn to family and friends for support.

Small Intestine

Cramps and gas are common symptoms of the diet, especially in the early stages. Back off probiotic foods, or consult your food journal to see what new food you recently added.

Skin Issues

The largest organ in your body, your skin is directly involved with detoxification. You might have temporary skin issues as your body rids itself of toxins by every available path.

Large Intestine

Diarrhea is another die-off symptom. Drink extra water or broth to replace your fluids. Constipation also is common. If you are prone, start with the full diet for 6 months.

Weight Loss

It's quite likely you'll lose weight on the diet. Many people who lose weight gain a bit when they go on the full GAPS diet before normalizing at a healthy weight.

DO	DON'T
✓ **Start slowly.** Spend 1 to 3 months on the full diet before starting the introduction stage, especially if your diet has been full of processed foods and sugar and lacking in nutrient-dense whole foods.	✗ **Jump right into the intro.** Give yourself at least a month to feel comfortable with making stock, broth, fermented vegetables, and cultured dairy before starting the intro diet. Source ingredients and tools before you begin.
✓ **Make time.** Plan on reducing your personal commitments for the duration of the intro diet. Part of the diet is providing your body with adequate rest so you can heal.	✗ **Start at the wrong time.** Right before the holiday season, a vacation, a big social event such as a wedding, or a big life change like a new job is not the time to begin the intro stage.
✓ **Talk about it.** Decide how you're going to talk to family and friends about your protocol. Often it's helpful to tell them you're on a temporary program that will help you with your uncomfortable symptoms.	✗ **Go out to eat.** Avoid dining out in early stages. In later stages, check the menu and come up with a plan, or call the restaurant ahead of time to see how they can accommodate your needs.
✓ **Take things slow and easy.** Most people spend 2 to 5 days at each stage. You can spend up to 7, after which it's time to move on, unless your digestive symptoms are still severe.	✗ **Force yourself to suffer.** If your die-off symptoms are too intense, reduce the amount of probiotic foods or supplements for a few days and then resume.
✓ **Support the detox process.** Brush your skin 5 minutes a day to stimulate your lymphatic system. Take 30-minute detox baths with 1 cup sea salt, baking soda, or apple cider vinegar in warm bath water.	✗ **Cheat for any reason.** Remind yourself of all you have to gain. Remember how uncomfortable your symptoms are.

Preparing Yourself

Ensuring your body and mind are in the right place before starting the healthy gut diet increases your chances of success. Follow this timeline to help get your body and mind in good shape.

3 to 6 Months Before

- Plan exactly when you want to start, ensuring your schedule is free from travel plans or special events you must attend.

- Begin to make healthier choices such as cutting sugar, grains, and soda.

- Eliminate any foods for which you suspect you have an allergy or intolerance.

- Begin using healthy fats for everyday cooking.

- Consider finding a buddy to go through the diet with you. Doing it with someone else is more fun and holds you accountable, which gives you a better chance of sticking with it.

- If you haven't already, read the book *Gut and Psychology Syndrome* by Dr. Natasha Campbell-McBride.

1 to 3 Months Before

- Experiment making one full-diet recipe per week, and build up to all full-diet meals and snacks.

- Source any supplements you'll be using on the diet.

- Source any cultures you'll need for dairy.

- Check in with your doctor about the diet. Find out which supplements and pharmaceuticals you must continue for the duration of the introduction diet.

- Consider finding a certified GAPS practitioner or online community for support.

- Begin to tell family and friends about your plan so you can gain their understanding and support.

- Mentally prepare for the diet. List the symptoms you want to stop, and write down how your life will change after you've healed.

2 Weeks Before

- Make sauerkraut, and store it in the refrigerator so you have fermented vegetable juice for stages 1 and 2.

- If necessary, order meat and bones from a local health food store or farmer.

- Resist the urge to binge one last time before you start!

1 Week Before

- Plan and shop for your first week of meals.

- Make large batches of stock, which you can use to cook soup. Freeze some, and store some in the refrigerator.

- If dairy isn't an issue for you, make yogurt or cultured cream for the first week.

Keeping a Food Journal

A food journal can be a powerful tool while you're going through the stages of the GAPS introduction. As you begin to add back foods to your diet, a food journal helps you detect any intolerances you may discover. It also helps you track your progress as you heal your leaky gut and make your way toward improved health.

DATE: January 15

Stage 1

Meal	Food	Beverage	Digestive Change	Mood Change
Breakfast	Chicken Vegetable Soup	24 oz (710ml) water, upon waking	Morning BM	Woke up rested
Snack	Butternut Squash Soup	16 oz (475ml) water, sipped throughout the morning	None	Alert, clear-headed
Lunch	Chicken Vegetable Soup	8 oz (240ml) water, 30 minutes before meal	None	None
Snack	Butternut Squash Soup	16 oz (475ml) water, sipped throughout the afternoon	None	slightly tired before meal (add more fat at lunch?)
Dinner	Lemon Peppercorn Poached Chicken Breast	8 oz (240ml) water, 30 minutes before meal	Gas, cramping (possible die-off?)	None
Snack	Butternut Squash Soup	8 oz (240ml) water, sipped throughout the evening	None	None

Preparing Your Kitchen and Pantry

Having the tools and ingredients you need for the healthy gut diet on hand before you begin makes everything go more smoothly when you start.

Sourcing Ingredients

Before you begin the diet, start to source your ingredients. Look for places to get grass-fed and pasture-raised meats, bones, animal fats, coconut oil, ghee, filtered water, and organic vegetables. For meats, bones, animal fats, and organic vegetables, try your local farmers' market. Check websites like eatwild.com or localharvest.org to find farmers who have healthy and sustainable practices. Health food stores are another option, although they might be more expensive. You should be able to find coconut oil, ghee, and filtered water at many local grocery or health food stores.

Making Ahead

You'll save time and make your life much easier if you cook some foods ahead of time:

- **Stocks and broths** Cook these ahead and store them in your refrigerator (up to 2 weeks if there's a solid layer of fat to preserve it) or freezer.

- **Soups** Create soups from the broths, and store for future meals.

- **Ferments and cultures** You need to start these 7 days before you plan on eating them. You'll need fermented juices for the early stages of the diet.

- **Ghee** You can make ghee from your own butter if you prefer not to use store-bought.

Finding Specialized Tools

In addition to the common cooking equipment you usually use—like measuring cups, knives, baking trays and dishes, and heavy-bottomed skillets—you'll find yourself making much use of more specialized kitchen equipment on the healthy gut diet:

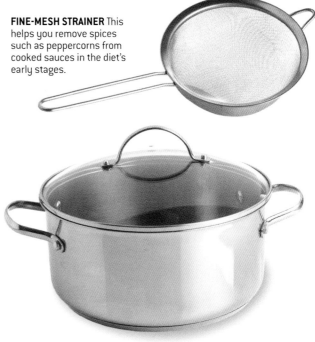

FINE-MESH STRAINER This helps you remove spices such as peppercorns from cooked sauces in the diet's early stages.

STOCKPOT This is an essential pan for making stocks, broths, and soups.

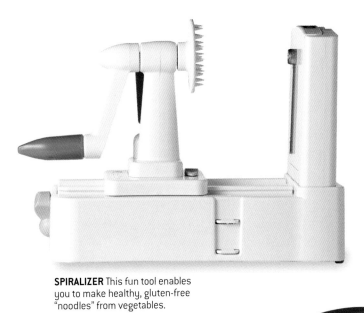

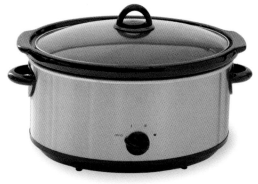

SPIRALIZER This fun tool enables you to make healthy, gluten-free "noodles" from vegetables.

SLOW COOKER This appliance is a handy alternative to making stocks, broths, and soups on the stove.

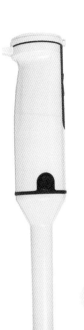

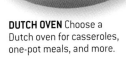

GLASS JARS You'll used these to store broths and stocks, as well as hold ferments and cultures.

DUTCH OVEN Choose a Dutch oven for casseroles, one-pot meals, and more.

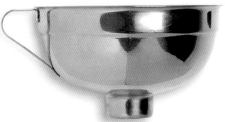

HAND BLENDER This appliance is handy for puréeing vegetables for smooth soups.

WIDE-MOUTH FUNNEL This is helpful for pouring stocks and cultures into jars for storage.

JUICER This appliance easily extracts juice from fruits and vegetables for making antioxidant-rich juice drinks.

Planning Ahead

When starting the healthy gut diet, you might feel overwhelmed by the new ingredients and techniques the protocol requires. But in a few weeks, or even a few days, these things will become familiar and even routine. In the meantime, developing a plan can help.

Planning Your Meals

- **Keep it simple** Especially in the earliest stages of the intro diet, opt for soup for most meals. Choose two or three for the week, and double the recipes, if necessary, to freeze individual portions.

- **Make ahead** In later stages, depending on your family or lifestyle, plan to cook three or four meals a week and save the rest for leftovers.

- **Get creative** Have breakfast for dinner or dinner for breakfast if you like.

Purchasing Ingredients

- **Stay local** Find a good source of whole chicken and beef bones, preferably pastured and grass-fed. Eatwild.com can help you locate local farmers, or you may be able to get what you need at your local health food store or farmers' market.

- **Choose quality** If you can't find grass-fed or pastured meats, buy the highest quality you can locate and afford. Many people have healed using what they find at their local grocery store.

- **Find healthy fats** Locate sources for coconut oil and butter and any other animal fat (such as lard) if possible. Health food stores and farmers' markets are good sources for these, too.

Cooking Ahead

- **Think about variety** Alternate soups so you don't get bored. Have one meat-based soup and one vegetable-based soup on hand so you can mix things up.

- **Reduce broths** When storing broth, you can reduce it so it takes up less space in your freezer. Simply let it boil until you have half or a quarter of the original volume. Be sure to label your jars so you remember how much water to add when you want to use it.

- **Stick to a schedule** Ferments take time. It's very important to stick to a schedule so you don't find yourself without veggies or cultured dairy.

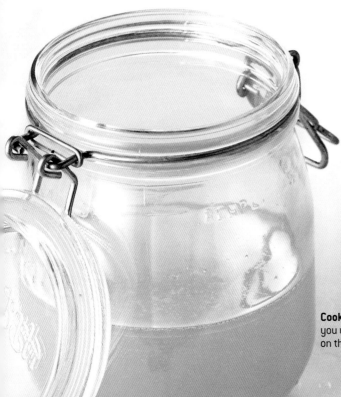

Cooking ahead sets you up for success on the diet.

Storing Food

- **Can in jars** The easiest way to store broth and soup is in glass canning jars, available at grocery or hardware stores. You can use these in the refrigerator or freezer. (Be sure to leave a head space at the top of the jar for the soup to expand if freezing.) Soup can last for several months in the freezer before it crystallizes.

- **Vacuum seal** If you have a vacuum sealer, you can use it to store soups in the freezer. Follow the manufacturer's instructions for storing liquids. Vacuum-sealed soup lasts for several months.

- **Freeze or refrigerate** Other foods can be refrigerated in glass or BPH-free plastic containers. If the soup has a thick cap of fat on top, it'll last up to 10 days.

Broths and soups can be stored in jars in your refrigerator or freezer.

SAVING MONEY

If you're on a budget, you have many options to consider for saving money on the diet:

- Your local farmers' market is a great source for less-expensive organic vegetables, meats, and fats.

- Ask for "seconds" when you shop. These are vegetables that aren't cosmetically perfect but offer the same nutritional value, often at a fraction of the cost.

- Try to choose vegetables in season when they're less expensive and easier to find.

- Grow some of your own vegetables. Even a few containers on your porch can yield a plentiful harvest.

- For meats and bones, consider buying a half- or quarter-cow from a local farmer, or split the order with a friend or family member. Buying direct and in bulk is a great way to economize.

- Keep your eyes open for sales, which are often seasonal and based on when animals are butchered. Keep in mind that bones are often very inexpensive.

- Making broth and stock-based soups helps you stretch your budget without sacrificing nutritional healing.

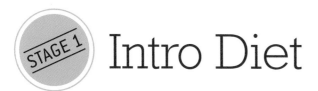

STAGE 1 Intro Diet

Welcome to the start of your journey! Beginning a diet protocol like this is a big step toward restoring your health. As you get started, be gentle with yourself. Keep things as simple as possible, and give yourself time to rest and heal.

How This Stage Works

- **Elimination** In the beginning, you'll eliminate major irritants, potential allergens, and possible sensitivities that might be contributing to your gut dysbiosis.

- **Microbiome** In stage 1, bad bacteria have lost their food source—sugar. As a result, they begin to starve and die and move out of your body.

- **Timing** Plan to spend 2 to 5 days at each stage. Some people spend as many as 7 days on a stage, but at that point, you should move on to the next stage unless your digestive symptoms are still severe.

What You Can Expect

- **Die-off** As bad bacteria die, they release toxins. These substances can cause gas, bloating, diarrhea, and cramping. The worst of these symptoms usually last only a few days. Be strong, rest as much as you need to, and keep in mind that this stage is only temporary and is the first step to regaining your health.

- **Adjustments** In stage 1, you're getting rid of foods you've always eaten. Embrace the idea of new staple foods, new routines, and new mind-sets.

- **Boredom** The foods in stage 1 are limited on purpose. Keeping things simple can mean you're eating the same meal over and over. Vary as much as you can while still making things easy on yourself.

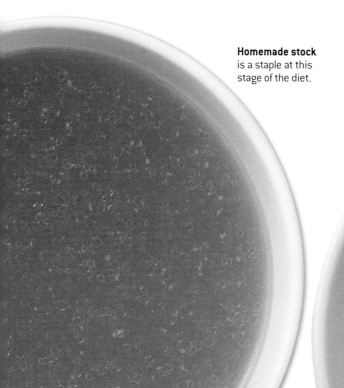

Homemade stock is a staple at this stage of the diet.

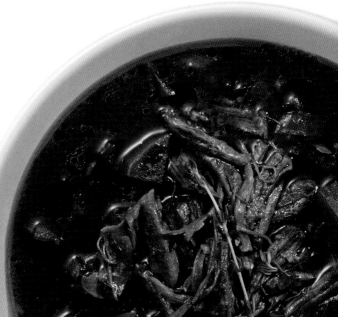

What You Can Eat

MEAT AND MEAT PRODUCTS These are the basis of this stage. Animal products are an important source of protein and fats, and they're rich in vitamins and minerals needed for gut healing.

- **Homemade stocks** Sip stocks made from beef, chicken, fish, turkey, and lamb between meals, or use as a base for soups. Grocery store stock is not the same and cannot be substituted.

- **Boiled meat** Your meat must be well boiled at this stage. Reserve meat, fat, and connective tissue from stock to use in other recipes.

- **Healthy fats** Use good fats such as tallow, lard, chicken, goose, or duck fat for cooking and in soups. Coconut oil also can be used. These fats are rich in the minerals that help heal your gut.

VEGETABLES AND VEGETABLE PRODUCTS You can eat vegetables if they're well cooked; don't eat fermented vegetables at this stage. All types of vegetables are healthy, but at this stage, avoid more fibrous vegetables to give your gut a rest.

- **Cooked vegetables** Vegetables must be well cooked and should be peeled. Avoid fibrous vegetables such as cabbage and asparagus, and remove fibrous parts such as the stems of cauliflower and broccoli.

- **Juice only** You can use only the juice of fermented vegetables at this stage; cabbage is too fibrous. Try adding 1 teaspoon to soup that's been cooled to lukewarm so the beneficial bacteria aren't killed.

> **TEA**
> To make tea, steep 1 tablespoon fresh ginger and 1 tablespoon fresh mint or 1 tablespoon organic loose-leaf chamomile tea in 1 cup boiling water for 5 or 6 minutes. Stir in 1 teaspoon raw honey, coconut oil, and/or fresh lemon juice to taste just before straining and serving.

CULTURED DAIRY This is allowed at this stage for those who have no allergy to it. For those who can tolerate it, dairy is a great vehicle for beneficial probiotics and a good source of protein and fats.

- **Cultured dairy** If you have no allergy to dairy, you can add homemade yogurt, cultured cream, or kefir (which have been cultured no less than 24 hours).

- **Homemade dairy** This is the only acceptable dairy during the intro stage. You can try commercial dairy later, when you're on the full GAPS diet.

- **Intolerance** If you suspect dairy intolerance, wait at least 6 months before attempting to reintroduce it.

SWEETENERS The only allowed sweeteners are raw honey, fruit (added in later stages), and whole-leaf stevia in small amounts. Stevia extract is not the same as whole-leaf stevia and should be avoided. Erythritol, sorbitol, and xylitol are all sugar alcohols that can cause gut issues because they're mostly indigestible.

Yogurt and other cultured dairy add probiotics (if you have no intolerence for dairy).

Beet and Beef Short Rib Borscht combines well-cooked vegetables and healing meat.

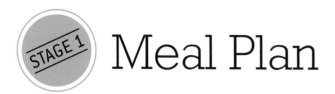

Meal Plan

STAGE 1

Time in the kitchen is essential for success with from-scratch, gut-healing recipes. Set aside time for planning before starting the diet or moving to the next stage so you can develop your kitchen skills and your shopping list.

NEW STAGE-SPECIFIC CHOICES and recommendations include the following:

- **Probiotic vegetable juice** Begin making a double batch of ferments at least 7 days before you start the diet. Save the vegetables to incorporate into later stages.

- **Probiotic dairy** If tolerated, begin making cultured dairy a few days before starting the protocol. Try Yogurt, Cultured Cream, or Kefir.

- **Homemade stock** Make a double batch of Chicken Stock and a single batch of Meat Stock 2 days before you begin so it's ready for sipping and for making soups. Plan to make extra to freeze. Add other stocks as your gut health improves.

- **Tea** Chamomile, mint, lemon, raw honey, whole-leaf stevia, and/or ginger.

- **Soup** Make two or three soups, with extra to freeze.

- **Entrées** Add one or more entrées for lunch or dinner later in your first week, and eat the leftovers for other meals. Try Beet and Beef Short Rib Borscht, Stewed Beef Porridge, and Lemon Peppercorn Poached Chicken Breast.

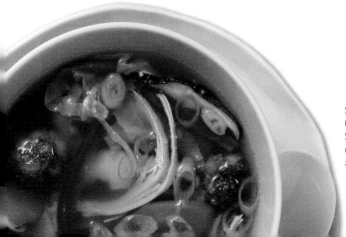

Sweet-and-Sour Chicken Vegetable Soup is a hearty comfort food for any meal.

	SUNDAY
BREAKFAST	Chicken Stock **Stage 1,** page 59
	Juice from Fermented Mixed Vegetables **Stage 1,** page 66
	Yogurt (optional) **Stage 1,** page 74
LUNCH	Chicken Stock **Stage 1,** page 59
	Juice from Fermented Mixed Vegetables **Stage 1,** page 66
	Yogurt (optional) **Stage 1,** page 74
DINNER	Chicken Stock **Stage 1,** page 59
	Juice from Fermented Mixed Vegetables **Stage 1,** page 66
	Yogurt (optional) **Stage 1,** page 74
SNACKS	Tea or homemade chicken, beef, or fish stock **Stage 1**

ONE-WEEK SAMPLE MEAL PLAN

MONDAY	TUESDAY	WEDNESDAY	THURSDAY	FRIDAY	SATURDAY
Chicken Stock **Stage 1,** page 59	Chicken Stock **Stage 1,** page 59	Meat Stock **Stage 1,** page 59	Chicken Stock **Stage 1,** page 59	Meat Stock **Stage 1,** page 59	Chicken Stock **Stage 1,** page 59
Juice from Fermented Mixed Vegetables **Stage 1,** page 66	Juice from Fermented Mixed Vegetables **Stage 1,** page 66	Juice from Fermented Mixed Vegetables **Stage 1,** page 66	Juice from Fermented Mixed Vegetables **Stage 1,** page 66	Juice from Fermented Mixed Vegetables **Stage 1,** page 66	Juice from Fermented Mixed Vegetables **Stage 1,** page 66
Yogurt (optional) **Stage 1,** page 74	Yogurt (optional) **Stage 1,** page 74	Yogurt (optional) **Stage 1,** page 74	Yogurt (optional) **Stage 1,** page 74	Yogurt (optional) **Stage 1,** page 74	Yogurt (optional) **Stage 1,** page 74
Chicken Stock **Stage 1,** page 59	Chicken Stock **Stage 1,** page 59	Classic Chicken Soup **Stage 1,** page 84	Carrot Beet Soup **Stage 1,** page 86	Three-Onion Soup **Stage 1,** page 93	Stewed Beef Porridge **Stage 1,** page 100
Juice from Fermented Mixed Vegetables **Stage 1,** page 66	Juice from Fermented Mixed Vegetables **Stage 1,** page 66	Juice from Fermented Mixed Vegetables **Stage 1,** page 66	Juice from Fermented Mixed Vegetables **Stage 1,** page 66	Juice from Fermented Mixed Vegetables **Stage 1,** page 66	Juice from Fermented Mixed Vegetables **Stage 1,** page 66
Yogurt (optional) **Stage 1,** page 74	Yogurt (optional) **Stage 1,** page 74	Yogurt (optional) **Stage 1,** page 74	Yogurt (optional) **Stage 1,** page 74	Yogurt (optional) **Stage 1,** page 74	Yogurt (optional) **Stage 1,** page 74
Chicken Stock **Stage 1,** page 59	Classic Chicken Soup **Stage 1,** page 84	Carrot Beet Soup **Stage 1,** page 86	Three-Onion Soup **Stage 1,** page 93	Stewed Beef Porridge **Stage 1,** page 100	Lemon Peppercorn Poached Chicken Breast **Stage 1,** page 101
Juice from Fermented Mixed Vegetables **Stage 1,** page 66	Juice from Fermented Mixed Vegetables **Stage 1,** page 66	Juice from Fermented Mixed Vegetables **Stage 1,** page 66	Juice from Fermented Mixed Vegetables **Stage 1,** page 66	Juice from Fermented Mixed Vegetables **Stage 1,** page 66	Juice from Fermented Mixed Vegetables **Stage 1,** page 66
Yogurt (optional) **Stage 1,** page 74	Yogurt (optional) **Stage 1,** page 74	Yogurt (optional) **Stage 1,** page 74	Yogurt (optional) **Stage 1,** page 74	Yogurt (optional) **Stage 1,** page 74	Yogurt (optional) **Stage 1,** page 74
Tea or homemade chicken, beef, or fish stock **Stage 1**	Tea or homemade chicken, beef, or fish stock **Stage 1**	Tea or homemade chicken, beef, or fish stock **Stage 1**	Tea or homemade chicken, beef, or fish stock **Stage 1**	Tea or homemade chicken, beef, or fish stock **Stage 1**	Tea or homemade chicken, beef, or fish stock **Stage 1**

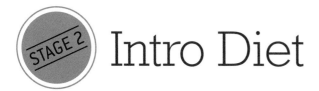

STAGE 2 Intro Diet

Stage 2 continues much in the same way as stage 1, with one big addition: eggs. Begin adding a raw egg yolk to a cup of soup, and increase until you're having two or three yolks with every cup of soup.

How This Stage Works

- **Some new, some old** Continue eating stage 1 foods while you add new stage 2 foods. You can still keep things simple and easy as you add some variety to your diet.

- **Slow progress** If you suspect an egg allergy might be to blame for any of your digestive issues, omit eggs for a day, see how you feel, and then try again. Use the same procedure for all new foods as you slowly add them to your diet.

- **Some relief** Keep going with the diet, and realize that even though you may have gotten relief from some of your symptoms, you aren't yet fully healed.

What You Can Expect

- **Die-off** Die-off should have slowed down or stopped by now, although you still might experience it in patches. Symptoms of die-off and allergy or intolerance to foods often can look the same, so consult your food journal as you add new foods to determine which is at play.

- **A healthy routine** Hopefully you've settled into a good groove with the diet by now. Stick to making stocks and soups, and now add stews.

- **Some improvement** You should be experiencing less gas, bloating, and discomfort, although much of that depends on where you started from in terms of symptoms.

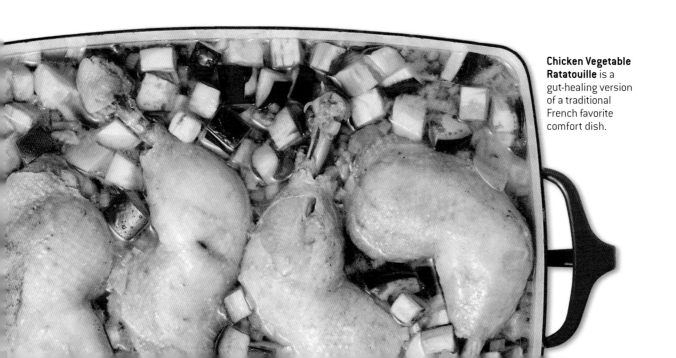

Chicken Vegetable Ratatouille is a gut-healing version of a traditional French favorite comfort dish.

What You Can Eat

STOCKS, SOUPS, AND STEWS These form the basis of stage 2 and are an easy and satisfying way to stay fueled. They also make your life much simpler because you're packing many gut-healing nutrients into an easy-to-heat-and-eat package.

- **Stocks and soups** Continue with stocks and soups, enjoying your favorites from stage 1.

- **Stews** You also can increase stews that have more meat and vegetables and less stock.

- **Boiled meats** Continue with meats that have been well boiled in soups, stews, or casseroles.

BOILED VEGETABLES AND FERMENTED JUICES

These are the best ways to enjoy your plant-based favorites at this stage. Boiling vegetables makes them easier to digest. It does remove some of the nutrients, so it's best to consume the water they were boiled is, such as with soup.

- **Boiled vegetables** Peeled, nonfibrous vegetables such as carrots, onions, beets, green beans, and broccoli (remove the fibrous stalks) that have been well boiled are easiest to tolerate.

- **Fermented vegetable juice** This continues to work well added to soups. Increase the amount, adjusting if the die-off reaction gets too intense.

> ### SEASONING AND SPICES
> For seasoning, use sea salt and peppercorns, removing the peppercorns before eating the finished dish. You also can use fresh herbs now. Rosemary, basil, tarragon, and sage are classics for soups. Tie them with kitchen twine to make them easy to remove from soups.

FATS AND DAIRY If tolerated, these still are great ways to get protein and nutrients in your diet. Many people who can't tolerate pasteurized and homogenized dairy can tolerate raw dairy, which allows them to enjoy the nutritional value without the digestive symptoms.

- **Animal fats and coconut oil** These healthy fats continue to be good additions.

- **Ghee** Ghee can be added at this stage. Begin with 1 teaspoon per day and gradually increase, watching for any intolerance.

- **Cod liver oil** This is another allowable addition at this stage. It's not for cooking but should be taken by the spoonful or in capsules. Check the GAPS website for recommendations.

- **Dairy products** If you tolerate them well, continue with dairy products. You can increase your servings at this stage.

Ghee is an essential fat you will use from this stage on, if you can tolerate dairy.

STAGE 2 Meal Plan

By now, you've probably started to get a handle on the ingredients and quantities to stock, how to prepare vegetables in bulk, and ways to store what you've produced. Stage 2 continues with much of the same, so keep building on your successes from stage 1 while also adding some new choices.

NEW STAGE-SPECIFIC CHOICES and recommendations include the following:

- **Probiotic vegetable juice** Try adding a fermentation you didn't make in stage 1 because the juice is still essential.

- **Dairy** Start with Home-Churned Butter, and use it to make the high-quality fat Ghee.

- **Homemade stocks** Continue with stocks you're already using, and add a batch or two of a new one. Choices include chicken, turkey, fish, beef, or lamb.

- **Soups** Try Egg Drop Soup and Vegetable Beef Stewp. Add fresh egg yolks to all your soups and stews for extra healing.

- **Entrées** New choices include Braised Beef (or turkey) Burgers, Asian Braised Turkey Meatballs, Ground Chicken Stuffed Cabbage Rolls, Chicken Vegetable Ratatouille, Chicken Enchilada Casserole, Lemon Rosemary Salmon, and Braised Tomato Sage Turkey Legs.

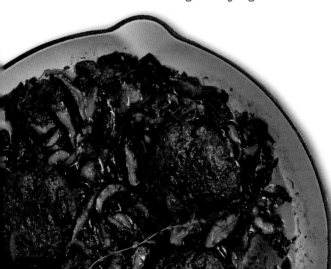

Braised Beef Burgers are a hearty way to enjoy ground meat with flavorful cooked vegetables.

SUNDAY

BREAKFAST

Chicken Stock
Stage 1, page 59

Juice from Fermented Mixed Vegetables
Stage 1, page 66

Yogurt (optional)
Stage 1, page 74

LUNCH

Butternut Squash Soup
Stage 1, page 85

Juice from Fermented Mixed Vegetables
Stage 1, page 66

Yogurt (optional)
Stage 1, page 74

DINNER

Braised Beef Burgers
Stage 2, page 108

Juice from Fermented Mixed Vegetables
Stage 1, page 66

Yogurt (optional)
Stage 1, page 74

SNACKS

Tea or homemade chicken, beef, or fish stock
Stage 1

ONE-WEEK SAMPLE MEAL PLAN

MONDAY	TUESDAY	WEDNESDAY	THURSDAY	FRIDAY	SATURDAY
Meat Stock **Stage 1,** page 58	Chicken Stock **Stage 1,** page 59	Meat Stock **Stage 1,** page 58	Chicken Stock **Stage 1,** page 59	Meat Stock **Stage 1,** page 58	Chicken Stock **Stage 1,** page 59
Juice from Fermented Mixed Vegetables **Stage 1,** page 66	Juice from Fermented Mixed Vegetables **Stage 1,** page 66	Juice from Fermented Mixed Vegetables **Stage 1,** page 66	Juice from Fermented Mixed Vegetables **Stage 1,** page 66	Juice from Fermented Mixed Vegetables **Stage 1,** page 66	Juice from Fermented Mixed Vegetables **Stage 1,** page 66
Yogurt (optional) **Stage 1,** page 74	Yogurt (optional) **Stage 1,** page 74	Yogurt (optional) **Stage 1,** page 74	Yogurt (optional) **Stage 1,** page 74	Yogurt (optional) **Stage 1,** page 74	Yogurt (optional) **Stage 1,** page 74
Egg Drop Soup **Stage 2,** page 106	Braised Beef Burgers **Stage 2,** page 108	Egg Drop Soup **Stage 2,** page 106	Creamy Tomato Soup **Stage 1,** page 96	Asian Braised Turkey Meatballs **Stage 2,** page 110	Lemon Rosemary Salmon **Stage 2,** page 115
Juice from Fermented Mixed Vegetables **Stage 1,** page 66	Juice from Fermented Mixed Vegetables **Stage 1,** page 66	Juice from Fermented Mixed Vegetables **Stage 1,** page 66	Juice from Fermented Mixed Vegetables **Stage 1,** page 66	Juice from Fermented Mixed Vegetables **Stage 1,** page 66	Juice from Fermented Mixed Vegetables **Stage 1,** page 66
Yogurt (optional) **Stage 1,** page 74	Yogurt (optional) **Stage 1,** page 74	Yogurt (optional) **Stage 1,** page 74	Yogurt (optional) **Stage 1,** page 74	Yogurt (optional) **Stage 1,** page 74	Yogurt (optional) **Stage 1,** page 74
Chicken Vegetable Ratatouille **Stage 2,** page 112	Butternut Squash Soup **Stage 1,** page 85	Chicken Vegetable Ratatouille **Stage 2,** page 112	Asian Braised Turkey Meatballs **Stage 2,** page 110	Lemon Rosemary Salmon **Stage 2,** page 115	Creamy Tomato Soup **Stage 1,** page 96
Juice from Fermented Mixed Vegetables **Stage 1,** page 66	Juice from Fermented Mixed Vegetables **Stage 1,** page 66	Juice from Fermented Mixed Vegetables **Stage 1,** page 66	Juice from Fermented Mixed Vegetables **Stage 1,** page 66	Juice from Fermented Mixed Vegetables **Stage 1,** page 66	Juice from Fermented Mixed Vegetables **Stage 1,** page 66
Yogurt (optional) **Stage 1,** page 74	Yogurt (optional) **Stage 1,** page 74	Yogurt (optional) **Stage 1,** page 74	Yogurt (optional) **Stage 1,** page 74	Yogurt (optional) **Stage 1,** page 74	Yogurt (optional) **Stage 1,** page 74
Tea or homemade chicken, beef, or fish stock **Stage 1**	Tea or homemade chicken, beef, or fish stock **Stage 1**	Tea or homemade chicken, beef, or fish stock **Stage 1**	Tea or homemade chicken, beef, or fish stock **Stage 1**	Tea or homemade chicken, beef, or fish stock **Stage 1**	Tea or homemade chicken, beef, or fish stock **Stage 1**

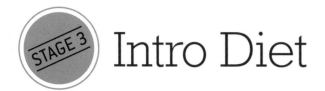

STAGE 3 Intro Diet

If, for the sake of convenience, you've been eating mostly soups for stages 1 and 2, stage 3 might feel like a revelation. Scrambled eggs for breakfast? Squash pancakes? Nut butter? It's a whole new world!

How This Stage Works

- **Gut calming** In stage 3, you're building on the progress you've made by calming your gut and removing reactive foods from your diet.

- **More good bacteria** You're continuing to make headway in controlling your gut's population of challenging bacteria, introducing more beneficial bacteria, and creating a more favorable environment for the bacteria to thrive.

- **New foods** You test the waters with new foods and become more deliberate about the inhabitants of your microbiome.

SUPPLEMENTS

During stage 3, you'll want to add a GAPS-legal therapeutic probiotic supplement. (For specific brand recommendations, consult the GAPS website.) But start slowly! Begin with a small dose, such as half a capsule, and gradually increase until you're taking the full dose.

What You Can Expect

- **Less digestive distress** By now, your digestive distress has probably calmed down quite a bit. Moving forward, any recurrence of symptoms is likely to be die-off, especially as you add probiotic foods.

- **Trial and error** If you have recurring digestive symptoms, you can step back to the preceding stage for a day and then move forward again. Alternatively, check your food diary to see what food you recently added, remove it, and see how your body responds.

- **Sensitivity testing** You can test a suspected food for sensitivity. If you don't show sensitivity, try reintroducing the food in a few weeks or even months. As your gut heals, you might be able to tolerate foods you never thought you'd be able to eat again.

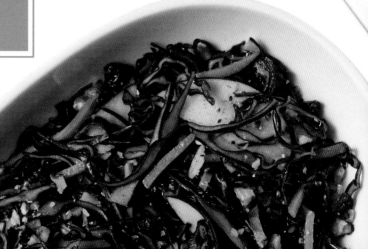

Sweet-and-Sour Red Slaw is a tasty way to enjoy fermented vegetables.

What You Can Eat

EGGS Cooked eggs in all their marvelous forms are a focus in this stage, providing protein and new textures. Eggs are delicious, and soft- and hard-boiled eggs make a convenient, portable snack.

- **Quality** Remember to find the highest-quality eggs possible.
- **Quantity** Plan on buying more than a dozen—you might find yourself eating eggs for breakfast, lunch, and dinner.
- **Cooking** Cook your eggs more gently at first, for example soft-boiled rather than hard-boiled. Use a lot of animal fat, coconut oil, or ghee when scrambling eggs.

Skillet Asparagus and Eggs is a delicious recipe to add back cooked eggs and vegetables to your diet.

FERMENTED VEGETABLES You can now eat the veggies instead of just the juice. There are two key words to remember as you begin: *start slowly.*

- **Start small** Try 1 or 2 teaspoons with a meal, and look for how your body responds. If your digestive symptoms recur with fermented vegetables, die-off is the likely culprit. Don't panic, and definitely don't lose hope. As uncomfortable as it can be, die-off is a good sign. You're making progress!
- **Small amounts** Reduce the amount of vegetables you're eating, even if that means you're only eating $1/2$ teaspoon of vegetables at a time.
- **Spread them out** You also can reduce the frequency, perhaps eating them with only one meal instead of all three.
- **Reduce symptoms** Do what you need to do to reduce your symptoms to a level you can live with. As your symptoms abate, increase the amount and frequency of vegetables until you're eating 1 or 2 tablespoons with each meal, listening to your body's responses carefully to set your pace.

HEALTHY FATS AND MORE In stage 3, you also add avocado and nut butter. Mash avocado to make simple guacamole, and eat nut butters on squash pancakes or simply off a spoon.

- **Start with almond butter** As always, go slowly and see how your body reacts. If you find that you react to one type of nut butter, try another.
- **Move beyond boiled vegetables** You now can add fully cooked (not just boiled) vegetables.
  - **Keep up the broth** Continue eating foods from stages 1 and 2 you enjoy. Sipping broth in the morning or between meals is still nourishing and healing to your gut.

STAGE 3 Meal Plan

You've made it to the halfway point in the introduction diet. More options now can mean more stress if you let it. Remember, you don't have to use every recipe available to you. It's fine to keep things simple. But bear in mind that including new recipes as you move forward helps you increase variety and best nourish your gut and body.

NEW STAGE-SPECIFIC CHOICES and recommendations include the following:

- **Probiotic vegetables** Red Cabbage Kraut and Sweet-and-Sour Red Slaw are two tasty ways to get your ferments.

- **Dairy** Continue including probiotic and cultured dairy as tolerated in your diet.

- **Hard-boiled eggs** This new addition is a satisfying, high-protein snack or meal.

- **Entrées** Try Sauerkraut Scramble, Santa Fe Breakfast Tostada, Skillet Asparagus and Eggs, Roasted Winter Squash Pancakes, Easy Avocado Omelet, and Aromatic Chicken with Mushrooms.

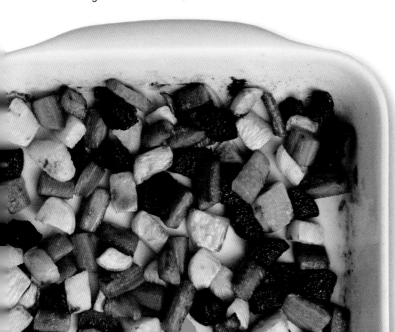

Simple Roasted Root Vegetables are great as a side with Aromatic Chicken with Mushrooms or on their own.

SUNDAY

BREAKFAST

Easy
Avocado Omelet
Stage 3, page 125

Fermented Mixed
Vegetables
Stage 1, page 66

LUNCH

Chicken
Vegetable Soup
Stage 1, page 88

DINNER

Roasted Winter
Squash Pancakes
Stage 3, page 124

Hard-boiled eggs
Stage 3

SNACKS

Tea or homemade
stock
Stage 1

ONE-WEEK SAMPLE MEAL PLAN

MONDAY	TUESDAY	WEDNESDAY	THURSDAY	FRIDAY	SATURDAY
Sauerkraut Scramble **Stage 3,** page 120	Skillet Asparagus and Eggs **Stage 3,** page 122 Red Cabbage Kraut **Stage 3,** page 64	Easy Avocado Omelet **Stage 3,** page 125 Fermented Mixed Vegetables **Stage 1,** page 66	Sauerkraut Scramble **Stage 3,** page 120	Skillet Asparagus and Eggs **Stage 3,** page 122 Red Cabbage Kraut **Stage 3,** page 64	Santa Fe Breakfast Tostada **Stage 3,** page 121 Fermented Mixed Vegetables **Stage 1,** page 66
Roasted Winter Squash Pancakes **Stage 3,** page 124 Hard-boiled eggs **Stage 3**	Garlicky Greens Soup **Stage 1,** page 89	Aromatic Chicken with Mushrooms **Stage 3,** page 126	Egg Drop Soup **Stage 2,** page 106	Braised Beef Burgers **Stage 2,** page 108	Egg Drop Soup **Stage 2,** page 106
Chicken Vegetable Soup **Stage 1,** page 88	Aromatic Chicken with Mushrooms **Stage 3,** page 126	Garlicky Greens Soup **Stage 1,** page 89	Braised Beef Burgers **Stage 2,** page 108	Egg Drop Soup **Stage 2,** page 106	Lemon Rosemary Salmon **Stage 2,** page 115
Tea or homemade stock **Stage 1**	Tea or homemade stock **Stage 1**	Tea or homemade stock **Stage 1**	Tea or homemade stock **Stage 1**	Tea or homemade stock **Stage 1**	Tea or homemade stock **Stage 1**

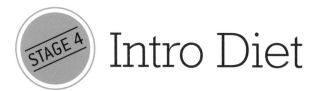

STAGE 4 Intro Diet

In stage 4, you'll start to feel like a normal person again who can eat (somewhat) normal food. The addition of baked and roasted meats and breads made from nut and seed flours brings a welcome variety.

How This Stage Works

- **New foods** As mentioned, you can enjoy new foods in stage 4. Add them slowly, paying attention to how your body reacts. Just because it's time to add a food to the protocol doesn't mean the food is right for you. Your body will show you. Gas, bloating, or diarrhea means you're not yet ready for that food.

- **Juice inclusion** At this stage, you can add some simple vegetable juices. Although beneficial, juicing is not strictly necessary, so if it's too much for you right now, set it aside and add it later.

- **Maintain** It's easy to feel like you've healed at this stage and can go back to your former habits. Don't!

What You Can Expect

- **Fewer symptoms** Most likely, your symptoms will have calmed down completely by now. You should be feeling increased energy and vitality.

- **More variety** Bread made with nut or seed flour gives you more options for meals during stage 4.

- **Dining out** Although eating out is more possible now, call ahead or check out the restaurant's menu online to be sure you can avoid prohibited ingredients, especially oils. Decide on menu options that will work for you before you get there.

Properly soaked and dried seeds, if you can tolerate them, are back on the menu. Or try seed flours for lots of new baking options.

Everyday Grain-Free Bread made with nut flours is a welcome reintroduction.

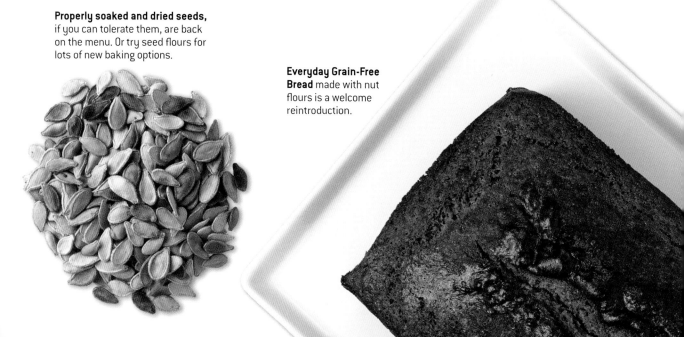

What You Can Eat

MEATS You have more options for preparing meat during this stage of the diet. You always can stick with your favorites from earlier stages, but now you have more variety available to you.

- **More choices** Beef, chicken, lamb, and fish are all good options, depending on your tastes.
- **Baking and roasting** These meat preparation methods are now allowed and add more flavor and texture to the finished dishes.
- **Barbecuing and frying** Avoid these preparation methods. They're still not allowed.

VEGETABLE JUICE At this stage of the diet, you can incorporate juice. This also gives you a way to promote detox. Now you can enjoy vegetable juices as a drink, but you need to work up to it.

- **Carrot juice** Begin slowly, with 1 teaspoon carrot juice per day on an empty stomach.
- **Celery, lettuce, and mint juices** Add these to your juicing protocol slowly. Find a combination you enjoy.
- **Don't go overboard.** Only drink a few tablespoons of juice at a time.

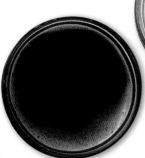
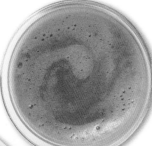

Vegetable juices return to your diet but need to be started slowly.

SUPPLEMENTS

Continue with your GAPS-legal probiotic. You also might need hydrochloric acid if your body doesn't produce enough and you have heartburn and acid indigestion. Take 1 betaine HCl tablet mid-meal, and increase by 1 tablet at each meal until you feel a warming sensation after taking the pills. Thereafter, take 1 fewer pill mid-meal as your dose, and monitor your reaction. Your dose might get lower as your health improves.

FATS Healthy fats are still a vital part of the diet, but now you have a popular new favorite to add back to your diet. But don't abandon the animal fats. They should be a permanent part of your diet.

- **Cold-pressed olive oil** You can use this fat now. Start sparingly and build up, watching your body for reactions.
- **Animal fats** Continue to use these for sautéing and in soups.
- **Canola, sunflower, and other vegetable oils** These are not permitted.

NUT FLOURS These bring a wealth of new choices. Now you can have gluten-free bread made with nut flours. Suddenly, sandwiches are back on the table, as are gluten-free empanadas and muffins.

- **Nut flour** You can use nut flours to make breads. Seed flour is also acceptable but probably best saved for later stages.
- **Almond flour** Start with almond flour, noticing how your body reacts. Progress slowly with other nut and seed flours. Nuts are often difficult to digest, so pay attention to what your body tells you.
- **Cashew or walnut flour** These are good choices for your next flour.

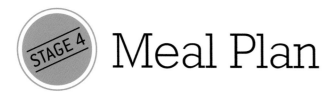

Meal Plan

STAGE 4

You've now hitting your stride! Having the options of roasting, baking, and grilling gives you a wider range of meat preparation techniques and flavors. Continue to keep things simple, but add variety when you can.

NEW STAGE-SPECIFIC CHOICES and recommendations include the following:

- **Probiotic vegetables** For increased variety, add the probiotic-rich Cultured Spring Vegetables, Cultured Root Vegetables, and Cultured Rainbow Vegetables ferments.

- **Dairy** Continue as tolerated.

- **Entrées** Use new ingredients and methods to create recipes you'll love, including Garlic Chicken with Vegetables, Grilled Salmon with Walnut Pesto, "Noodles" with Pomodoro Sauce, Oven-Roasted Turkey Meatloaf, Classic Pot Roast with Onions, Ground Beef Stroganoff, and Ground Beef Empanadas.

- **Snacks** Stocks and tea are still available as snacks, but adding some options will give you snack variety. Make a double batch of Ginger Pumpkin Muffins or Chicken Muffins, and freeze some for later. Or prep extra vegetables for Green Goddess Juice, Liver-Loving Juice, or Peppery Pear Juice ahead of time. Crackling Nuts or Crackling Seeds offer a satisfying crunch.

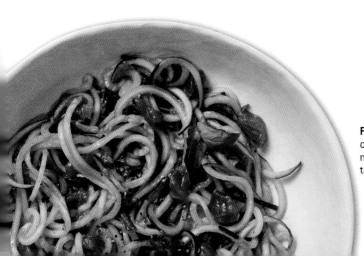

Flavorful sauces combine with "noodles" made from zucchini for tasty grain-free options.

SUNDAY

BREAKFAST

Carrot juice
Stage 4

Easy
Avocado Omelet
Stage 3, page 125

LUNCH

Carrot Beet Soup
Stage 1, page 86

DINNER

Classic Pot Roast
with Onions
Stage 4, page 139

SNACKS

Homemade beef
or chicken stock
Stage 1

Tea
Stage 1

Crackling Nuts
Stage 4, page 143

ONE-WEEK SAMPLE MEAL PLAN

MONDAY	TUESDAY	WEDNESDAY	THURSDAY	FRIDAY	SATURDAY
Carrot juice **Stage 4**	Carrot juice **Stage 4**	Carrot juice **Stage 4**	Carrot or vegetable juice **Stage 4**	Liver-Loving Juice **Stage 4,** page 133	Liver-Loving Juice **Stage 4,** page 133
Roasted Winter Squash Pancakes **Stage 3,** page 124	Sauerkraut Scramble **Stage 3,** page 120	Roasted Winter Squash Pancakes **Stage 3,** page 124	Chicken Muffins **Stage 4,** page 131	Roasted Winter Squash Pancakes **Stage 3,** page 124	Chicken Muffins **Stage 4,** page 131
Classic Pot Roast with Onions **Stage 4,** page 139	Carrot Beet Soup **Stage 1,** page 86	Vegetable Beef Stewp **Stage 2,** page 107	"Noodles" with Pomodoro Sauce **Stage 4,** page 136	Ground Beef Empanadas **Stage 4,** page 142	Oven-Roasted Turkey Meatloaf **Stage 4,** page 138
Vegetable Beef Stewp **Stage 2,** page 107	"Noodles" with Pomodoro Sauce **Stage 4,** page 136	Ground Beef Empanadas **Stage 4,** page 142	Oven-Roasted Turkey Meatloaf **Stage 4,** page 138	Skillet Asparagus and Eggs **Stage 3,** page 122	Aromatic Chicken with Mushrooms **Stage 3,** page 126
					Simple Roasted Root Vegetables **Stage 3,** page 127
Homemade beef or chicken stock **Stage 1**	Homemade beef or chicken stock **Stage 1**	Homemade beef or chicken stock **Stage 1**	Homemade beef or chicken stock **Stage 1**	Homemade beef or chicken stock **Stage 1**	Homemade beef or chicken stock **Stage 1**
Tea **Stage 1**	Tea **Stage 1**	Tea **Stage 1**	Tea **Stage 1**	Tea **Stage 1**	Tea **Stage 1**
Crackling Nuts **Stage 4,** page 143	Crackling Nuts **Stage 4,** page 143	Crackling Nuts **Stage 4,** page 143	Crackling Nuts **Stage 4,** page 143	Crackling Nuts **Stage 4,** page 143	Crackling Nuts **Stage 4,** page 143

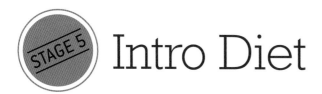

STAGE 5 Intro Diet

With the introduction of raw vegetables and spices in stage 5, you'll feel like your diet, and your life, is getting back to normal. Fruit also makes a limited appearance now, and after going so long with so little flavor, you'll find they taste amazingly sweet.

How This Stage Works

- **Some old, some new** Continue with the foods from past stages you still enjoy. You don't have to abandon those recipes just because you've moved on. Continue to enjoy your core favorites.

- **Increased juicing** Expand the foods you juice to include fruits as well as vegetables. Always aim for a higher percentage of vegetable juice.

- **Dish diversity** Experiment with new recipes, and enjoy the variety of dishes you can prepare and eat now. Also enjoy the fresher flavors of fruits and vegetables again.

What You Can Expect

- **Progress slowly** It can be easy at later stages to want to race ahead. But when adding new foods, do it slowly. Going too quickly could cause a setback.

- **Watch your reactions** Healing a leaky gut doesn't mean you can tolerate all foods. If your body reacts negatively to an added food, eliminate that food. Listen to your body.

- **Enjoy your progress** You have more energy now, and it's likely that you're very happy with what you see in the mirror and on the scale. Celebrate your success!

> **SPICES AND SEASONING**
> Some dried spices are allowed now. Start with peppercorns, basil, sage, thyme, parsley, ginger, cumin, coriander, paprika, and cloves. You add more spices in stage 6 and on the full GAPS diet.

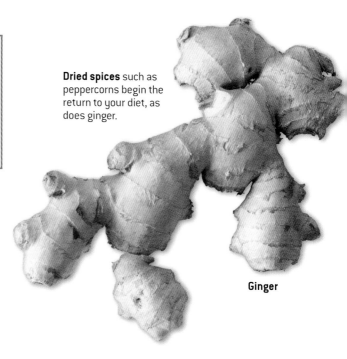

Dried spices such as peppercorns begin the return to your diet, as does ginger.

Ginger

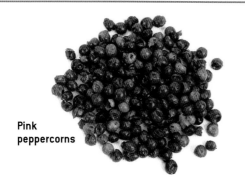

Pink peppercorns

What You Can Eat

RAW VEGETABLES These can now be incorporated in your diet. You'll enjoy their crisp freshness and bright flavors. Finally, you've worked your way up to raw vegetables, and that opens the door for salads.

- **Bring on the salad** Raw vegetables are now allowed. Salads of all sizes, flavors, and colors are a welcome change.

- **Start slowly** As always, start gently with soft lettuce and peeled cucumber.

- **Progress gradually** If you tolerate soft lettuce and peeled cucumber, progress to carrot, tomato, onion, and even cabbage, watching your body's responses.

FRUIT JUICES Fresh fruit juice is back on your menu, as are apples. The latter's delicious, juicy flesh adds natural sweetness to your meals.

- **Fruit juice** In addition to vegetable juice, you also can juice some fruits. Be sure you're keeping track of your juices in your food journal so you can detect any possible sensitivities.

- **Apple, mango, and pineapple juices** You can mix these juices with your vegetable juice. Make the fruit component no more than 20 to 25 percent of the mixture. No citrus fruits (other than lemon water) are allowed at this stage.

- **Baked apples** These are a delicious choice for dessert. Try them with cloves for a comforting fall flavor.

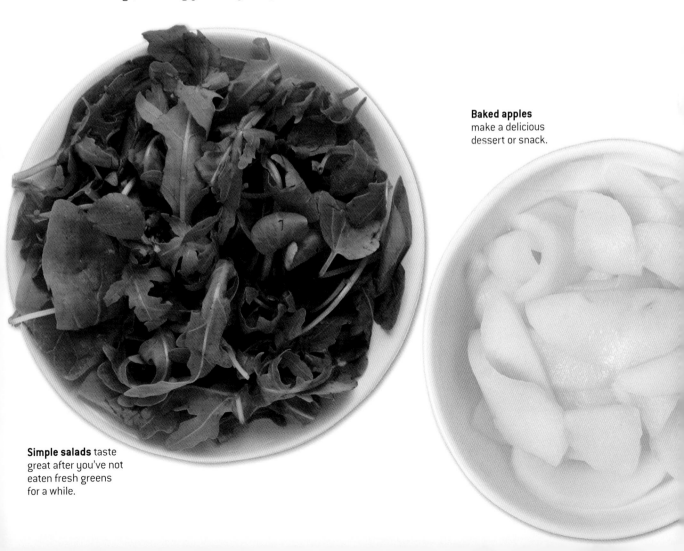

Baked apples make a delicious dessert or snack.

Simple salads taste great after you've not eaten fresh greens for a while.

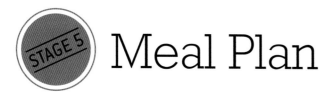

Meal Plan

STAGE 5

Stage 5 presents new ingredient opportunities. Fruits broaden your menu and bring naturally semisweet treats and more juices. Raw vegetables offer options for cold-prepped dishes, like salads, that give you a break from cooking.

NEW STAGE-SPECIFIC CHOICES and recommendations include the following:

- **Probiotic vegetables** Keep your ferments going! By stage 5, you've likely hit your stride with quantities and timing.

- **Dairy** Continue as tolerated.

- **Entrées** Incorporate new choices as you're able to keep things interesting and varied. Make ahead what you can when you can. Try Simple House Salad, Grain-Free Tabbouleh, Easy Chicken Stir-Fry, and Tex-Mex Pulled Pork Burritos.

- **Snacks** Snacks are important because they nourish you between meals and prevent hunger—plus, they're easy to make. Try Mini Butternut Squash Soufflés or Guacamole.

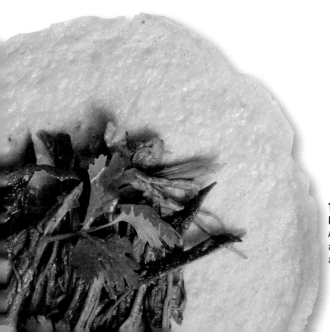

Tex-Mex Pulled Pork Burritos served on Almond Flour Wraps are zesty, festive, and healing.

	SUNDAY
BREAKFAST	Liver-Loving Juice **Stage 4,** page 133
	Skillet Asparagus and Eggs **Stage 3,** page 122
LUNCH	Grain-Free Tabbouleh **Stage 5,** page 147
	Pumpkin Bisque **Stage 1,** page 94
DINNER	Grilled Salmon with Walnut Pesto **Stage 4,** page 135
SNACKS	Liver-Loving Juice **Stage 4,** page 133
	Apple Pie Stewed Apples **Stage 5,** page 154
	Tea or homemade stock **Stage 1**

ONE-WEEK SAMPLE MEAL PLAN

MONDAY	TUESDAY	WEDNESDAY	THURSDAY	FRIDAY	SATURDAY
Vegetable juice **Stage 1** Easy Avocado Omelet **Stage 3**, page 125	Liver-Loving Juice **Stage 4**, page 133 Sauerkraut Scramble **Stage 3**, page 120	Liver-Loving Juice **Stage 4**, page 133 Skillet Asparagus and Eggs **Stage 3**, page 122	Green Goddess Juice **Stage 4**, page 132 Easy Avocado Omelet **Stage 3**, page 125	Liver-Loving Juice **Stage 4**, page 133 Sauerkraut Scramble **Stage 3**, page 120	Vegetable juice **Stage 1** Santa Fe Breakfast Tostada **Stage 3**, page 121
Simple House Salad **Stage 5**, page 146 Chicken Vegetable Soup **Stage 1**, page 88	Grain-Free Tabbouleh **Stage 5**, page 147 Pumpkin Bisque **Stage 1**, page 94	Simple House Salad **Stage 5**, page 146 Chicken Vegetable Soup **Stage 1**, page 88	Tex-Mex Pulled Pork Burritos with Almond Flour Wraps **Stage 5**, page 152	Asian Braised Turkey Meatballs **Stage 2**, page 110	Chicken Vegetable Ratatouille **Stage 2**, page 112
Easy Chicken Stir-Fry **Stage 5**, page 151	Lemon Peppercorn Poached Chicken Breast **Stage 1**, page 101	Tex-Mex Pulled Pork Burritos with Almond Flour Wraps **Stage 5**, page 152	Asian Braised Turkey Meatballs **Stage 2**, page 110	Chicken Vegetable Ratatouille **Stage 2**, page 112	Easy Chicken Stir-Fry **Stage 5**, page 151
Green Goddess Juice **Stage 4**, page 132 Chicken Muffins **Stage 4**, page 131 Tea or homemade stock **Stage 1**	Peppery Pear Juice **Stage 4**, page 132 Crackling Nuts **Stage 4**, page 143 Tea or homemade stock **Stage 1**	Liver-Loving Juice **Stage 4**, page 133 Baked Cinnamon Walnut Apples **Stage 5**, page 155 Tea or homemade stock **Stage 1**	Green Goddess Juice **Stage 4**, page 132 Guacamole **Stage 5**, page 150 Tea or homemade stock **Stage 1**	Peppery Pear Juice **Stage 4**, page 132 Mini Butternut Squash Soufflés **Stage 5**, page 148 Tea or homemade stock **Stage 1**	Liver-Loving Juice **Stage 4**, page 133 Hard-boiled eggs **Stage 3** Tea or homemade stock **Stage 1**

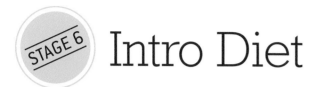

STAGE 6 Intro Diet

Congratulate yourself for all the hard work you've put in! As you complete this last stage of the introduction diet, you should reflect on where you started and how far you've come.

How This Stage Works

- **Increased honey, fruit, and whole-leaf stevia** As you begin to add more honey and fruit, pay careful attention to how your body responds; people can tolerate different amounts of these foods without blood sugar disruptions or weight gain. Whole-leaf stevia doesn't always adversely affect blood sugar, so if you're using it as your primary sweetener, you may not have any issues.

- **More nut consumption** Nuts aren't always easy to digest, even for a healthy gut. As you add more, especially in baked goods, watch for any increase in symptoms and remove the foods that cause trouble.

- **Moderation** This is an important rule to observe moving forward. If a new food works for you, don't go overboard. Binging is not a healthy behavior and doesn't contribute to gut health.

What You Can Expect

- **More sweets** As long as honey or whole-leaf stevia are the sweeteners, you can have more sweets now. Carefully watch how your body responds, though. If your digestive symptoms return, or if your blood sugar swings, back off the sweets.

- **Weight loss** Some weight loss is normal on the GAPS protocol. If you're concerned you've lost too much weight, wait to see what happens when you go onto the full GAPS diet. Most people find a new, healthy normal once they've been on the full diet.

- **Sense of accomplishment** This is totally appropriate. You've shown great patience and restraint. Great job!

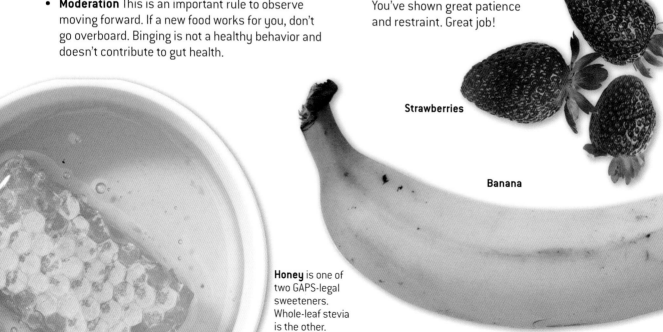

Strawberries

Banana

Honey is one of two GAPS-legal sweeteners. Whole-leaf stevia is the other.

What You Can Eat

RAW FRUITS Finally, you should be able to tolerate raw fruit now. Add fruit back to your diet slowly and watchfully, starting with these.

- **Raw fruit** Slowly add more raw fruit from the list of GAPS-approved foods.

- **Berries** With their high fiber content, berries are a great place to start.

- **Canned or preserved fruits** Jams or jellies are not allowed. Stick to whole or diced fruits with lower sugar.

SWEETENED FOODS With honey or whole-leaf stevia as the sweetener, these treats can make a return to your diet. Still, be cautious as you slowly reintroduce these foods. After so long without them, they might taste too sweet right now.

- **Experiment with more honey** If you do well with it, you can increase your honey intake. Watch for any carbohydrate sensitivity, such as mood and energy swings, weight gain, or binge behavior.

- **Desserts** These can be increased during stage 6. Again, watch for any sensitivity.

- **Taste changes** Your taste buds likely have recalibrated so you can taste the complex sweetness of dishes.

NUTS Brazil nuts can be added at this stage. As with other foods you reintroduce, be aware of any digestive symptoms you experience and back off as necessary.

Fresh fruit is a healthy way to add some sweetness to your diet. Berries especially are rich in fiber and antioxidants.

Raspberries

Blueberries

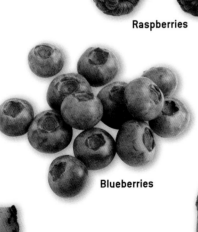

Seasonal Mixed-Berry Crostata combines luscious seasonal fruits with a gluten-free crust.

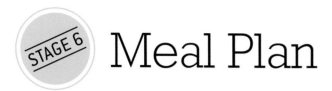

STAGE 6 Meal Plan

You've made it to stage 6 of the intro diet. You're more confident in the kitchen and making only small tweaks to your overall plan. Now a few new ingredients and tasty recipes help keep you healthy and enthusiastic as you head toward the full diet.

NEW STAGE-SPECIFIC CHOICES and recommendations include the following:

- **Probiotic vegetables** Keep your ferments going, and look for your own recipe variations.

- **Dairy** Continue as tolerated.

- **Entrées** New entrée options let you tailor your plan to your family preferences. Try Roasted Brussels Sprout Apple Salad, Scallops Piccata, and Chicken Thigh Puttanesca.

- **Desserts** High-quality homemade desserts are a satisfying and appropriate part of gut health. Try Dairy-Free Key Lime Mousse, Seasonal Mixed-Berry Crostada, Honey Bombs, and Gingered Vanilla Honey Drops.

- **Snacks** Extra snack recipes keep you satisfied throughout the day. Try an Anytime Smoothie or the Olive Raisin Tapenade, which is great as a dip or a topping for roasted meat.

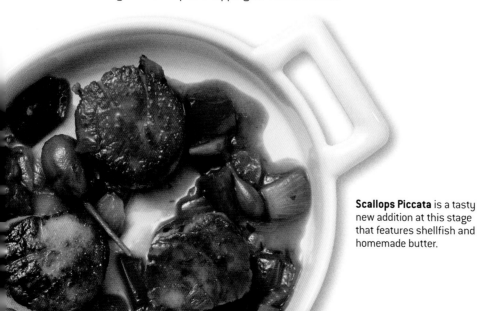

Scallops Piccata is a tasty new addition at this stage that features shellfish and homemade butter.

SUNDAY

BREAKFAST

Peppery
Pear Juice
Stage 4, page 132

Easy
Avocado Omelet
Stage 3, page 125

LUNCH

Simple
House Salad
Stage 5, page 146

Creamy
Tomato Soup
Stage 1, page 96

DINNER

Scallops Piccata
Stage 6, page 160

SNACKS

Seasonal
Mixed-Berry
Crostata
Stage 6, page 166

Chicken Muffins
Stage 4, page 131

ONE-WEEK SAMPLE MEAL PLAN

MONDAY	TUESDAY	WEDNESDAY	THURSDAY	FRIDAY	SATURDAY
Roasted Winter Squash Pancakes **Stage 3,** page 124	Green Goddess Juice **Stage 4,** page 132	Liver-Loving Juice **Stage 4,** page 133	Green Goddess Juice **Stage 4,** page 132	Peppery Pear Juice **Stage 4,** page 132	Santa Fe Breakfast Tostada **Stage 3,** page 121
Liver-Loving Juice **Stage 4,** page 133	Sauerkraut Scramble **Stage 3,** page 120	Skillet Asparagus and Eggs **Stage 3,** page 122	Easy Avocado Omelet **Stage 3,** page 125	Sauerkraut Scramble **Stage 3,** page 120	
Beet and Beef Short Rib Borscht **Stage 1,** page 98	Roasted Brussels Sprout Apple Salad **Stage 6,** page 159	Beet and Beef Short Rib Borscht **Stage 1,** page 98	Chicken Thigh Puttanesca **Stage 6,** page 163	Braised Beef Burgers **Stage 2,** page 108	Ground Chicken Stuffed Cabbage Rolls **Stage 2,** page 111
	Three-Onion Soup **Stage 1,** page 93				
Pan Steak with Mushrooms **Stage 1,** page 102	Chicken Thigh Puttanesca **Stage 6,** page 163	Braised Beef Burgers **Stage 2,** page 108	Roasted Winter Squash Pancakes **Stage 3,** page 124	Ground Chicken Stuffed Cabbage Rolls **Stage 2,** page 111	Roasted Brussels Sprout Apple Salad **Stage 6,** page 159
			Scrambled eggs **Stage 3**		Three-Onion Soup **Stage 1,** page 93
Dairy-Free Key Lime Mousse **Stage 6,** page 164	Honey Bombs **Stage 6,** page 168	Baked Cinnamon Walnut Apples **Stage 5,** page 155	Olive Raisin Tapenade **Stage 6,** page 162	Anytime Smoothie **Stage 6,** page 158	Gingered Vanilla Honey Drops **Stage 6,** page 169
Peppery Pear Juice **Stage 4,** page 132	Anytime Smoothie **Stage 6,** page 158	Green Goddess Juice **Stage 4,** page 132	Guacamole **Stage 5,** page 150	Apple Pie Stewed Apples **Stage 5,** page 154	Crackling Nuts **Stage 4,** page 143

The Full Diet

FULL DIET

You've made it through the introduction diet. Not only are you feeling better, but you're also reaping the rewards of a healthy gut, ranging from hormone balance, to reduced inflammation, to better emotional and mental well-being.

How This Stage Works

- **Expanded menu** On the full diet, your food choices are greater. Visit gapsdiet.com for specifics on what you can eat and what you should continue to avoid.

- **Balance** Take it easy on desserts and starchier carbs. Your microbiome is delicately balanced, and too much of anything can give opportunistic bacteria the upper hand.

- **Symptom control** You can repeat the introduction diet once a year or whenever you feel symptoms beginning to reoccur.

What You Can Expect

- **New foods** Take care when adding new foods, maintain your food journal, and wait a few days between additions to see how your body responds.

- **Plan ahead** Before going out to eat or to a party, have an idea what you can eat. Be sure there's something acceptable for you to eat so you don't jeopardize your healing.

- **Temptation** Wanting to eat foods that aren't GAPS legal is normal. Remember where you came from, and stay strong. If you go back to eating the way you used to eat, you'll eventually find yourself right back where you started.

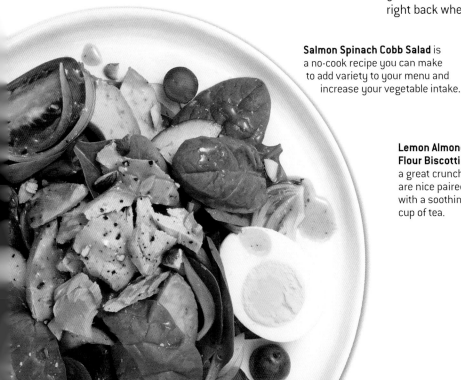

Salmon Spinach Cobb Salad is a no-cook recipe you can make to add variety to your menu and increase your vegetable intake.

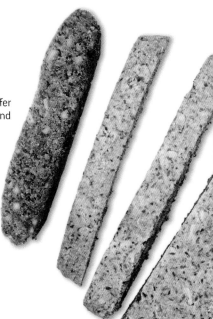

Lemon Almond Flour Biscotti offer a great crunch and are nice paired with a soothing cup of tea.

What You Can Eat

VEGETABLES Cooked and raw vegetables are now a bigger part of your diet. More fibrous vegetables also make a comeback as your range increases.

- **Versatile veggies** Add back rutabagas, rhubarb, eggplant, and bell peppers, as well as seaweed.
- **Some beans and legumes** Try lentils, navy beans, lima beans, split peas, peanuts, and peanut butter.

FRUITS Your range of fruits is much greater now, and you can enjoy stronger flavors and textures.

- **Citrus** Add kumquats, grapefruit, limes, oranges, tangerines, and satsumas.
- **Tropical fruits** Liven up your meals with mangoes, pineapple, and papaya.
- **Favorites** Other fruits also return for snacking and sides, such as melons, grapes, and even olives.

DAIRY If you tolerate it, dairy is another expanded category with a variety of more complex cheeses.

- **Deli favorites** Now you can enjoy colby, Swiss, Monterey Jack, and Muenster cheeses.
- **Table cheeses** Havarti, edam, and gouda slice and melt well and can boost the flavor of your meals.
- **Harder cheeses** Asiago and Romano grate well and can expand your salad horizons.
- **Softer, stronger cheeses** Bleu cheese, gorgonzola, limburger, camembert, Port du Salut, Stilton, and Roquefort now can be part of your menu.

> ### SUPPLEMENTS
> Continue with probiotics, cod liver oil, HCl, and ox bile (if you need it), adjusting as necessary. You also can work with a certified GAPS practitioner if you think you need help fine-tuning your supplements.

ALCOHOL On occasion, small amounts of alcohol are allowable now. One drink at a celebratory occasion is one thing; a cocktail every night can cause a relapse. Explore naturally fermented beverages like kombucha that help maintain gut health instead of disturbing it.

- **Liquor** You can enjoy an occasional cocktail with gin or a shot of scotch.
- **Wine** A glass of dry red or white wine with a meal now and then is allowed.

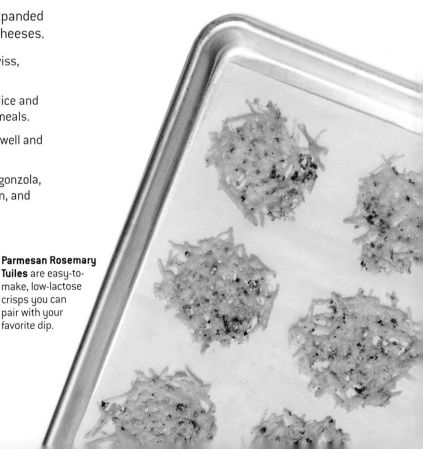

Parmesan Rosemary Tuiles are easy-to-make, low-lactose crisps you can pair with your favorite dip.

Meal Plan

FULL DIET

You're now full GAPS legal, but it's no time to get complacent. To maintain your gut health progress, it's important to keep moving forward. Focus on increasing variety as you plan your meals, continue to challenge your kitchen skills, and maximize your nutrient intake potential to nourish your gut and body.

NEW STAGE-SPECIFIC CHOICES and recommendations include the following:

- **Probiotic vegetables** Kimchi and Kowabunga Kimchi are new recipes for your fermenting arsenal.

- **Dairy** Continue as tolerated.

- **Entrées** Don't be overwhelmed by the number of new choices. Remember what you've learned about planning and preparing, and incorporate a few at a time into your menu.

- **Desserts** In moderation, semisweet options like Spiced Carrot Cake, Very Berry "Ice Cream," and Lemon Almond Flour Biscotti go a long way toward satisfying a sweet tooth.

- **Snacks** Pick a few each week to focus on. Spreads and dips can double as sauces and condiments. New choices include Hunger Buster Bars, Nut Butter, Nut Cheese, Parmesan Rosemary Tuiles, Three-Seed Crackers, Cauliflower Hummus, Roasted Eggplant Spread, Garden Fresh Salsa, and Tzatziki Sauce.

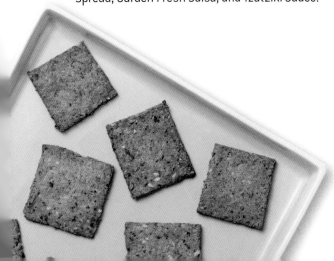

Three-Seed Crackers are a crunchy snack you can enjoy with chicken salad or your favorite nut or dairy cheese.

	SUNDAY
BREAKFAST	Grilled Vegetable Frittata **Full diet,** page 177
LUNCH	Calming Kale Salad **Full diet,** page 180
	Creamy Tomato Soup **Stage 1,** page 96
DINNER	Shrimp and Cauliflower Grits **Full diet,** page 199
SNACKS	Tea or stock **Stage 1**
	Very Berry "Ice Cream" **Full diet,** page 212
	Lemon Almond Flour Biscotti **Full diet,** page 214

ONE-WEEK SAMPLE MEAL PLAN

MONDAY	TUESDAY	WEDNESDAY	THURSDAY	FRIDAY	SATURDAY
Grainless Granola **Full diet,** page 176 Nut Milk **Stage 4,** page 71	Grilled Vegetable Frittata **Full diet,** page 177	Grainless Granola **Full diet,** page 176 Nut Milk **Stage 4,** page 71	Sausage, Egg, and Cheese Sandwich **Full diet,** page 173	Grainless Granola **Full diet,** page 176 Nut Milk **Stage 4,** page 71	Cheddar Chive Biscuits with Sausage Gravy **Full diet,** page 174
Grilled Vegetable Frittata **Full diet,** page 177	Chopped Cobb Salad **Full diet,** page 178 Creamy Tomato Soup **Stage 1,** page 96	Oven-Roasted Moroccan Chicken with Morrocan Cauliflower "Couscous" **Full diet,** page 196	Tuna Cakes with Rémoulade **Full diet,** page 195 Slammin' Hot Slaw **Full diet,** page 198	Vegetable Beef Stewp **Stage 2,** page 107	Margherita Pizza **Full diet,** page 194
Lamb Burger Sliders **Full diet,** page 192 Kimchi **Full diet,** page 200	Oven-Roasted Moroccan Chicken with Morrocan Cauliflower "Couscous" **Full diet,** page 196	Tuna Cakes with Rémoulade **Full diet,** page 195 Slammin' Hot Slaw **Full diet,** page 198	Vegetable Beef Stewp **Stage 2,** page 107	Margherita Pizza **Full diet,** page 194	Skillet Asparagus and Eggs **Stage 3,** page 122
Tea or stock **Stage 1** Nut Butter, Nut Cheese, or dairy cheese with Three-Seed Crackers **Full diet,** pages 208, 209, 206 Green Goddess Juice **Stage 4,** page 132	Tea or stock **Stage 1** Hunger Buster Bars **Full diet,** page 211 Anytime Smoothie **Stage 6,** page 158	Tea or stock **Stage 1** Roasted Eggplant Spread with Parmesan Rosemary Tuiles **Full diet,** pages 202, 204 Baked Cinnamon Walnut Apples **Stage 5,** page 155	Tea or stock **Stage 1** Liver-Loving Juice **Stage 4,** page 133 Seasonal Mixed-Berry Crostada **Stage 6,** page 166	Tea or stock **Stage 1** Hunger Buster Bars **Full diet,** page 211 Olive Raisin Tapenade **Stage 6,** page 162 Parmesan Rosemary Tuiles **Full diet,** page 204	Tea or stock **Stage 1** Peppery Pear Juice **Stage 4,** page 132 Cauliflower Hummus **Full diet,** page 202 Three-Seed Crackers **Full diet,** page 206

Going Forward

After transitioning into the full GAPS diet, many people wonder when they can go back to their old way of eating. The short answer is, never. The full GAPS diet is intended to become your everyday way of eating. Once dysbiosis has been established in your gut, you'll generally always need to avoid certain foods like refined sugars and grain, especially if you had a severe condition. The good news is that there are many more foods you can eat compared to those you can't eat. Here are a few things to keep in mind as you move forward.

Milestone 1 The 80/20 Rule

3 TO 6 MONTHS INTO THE DIET Most people try to shoot for 80 percent GAPS, 20 percent "cheating" in their menu. Keep in mind, if you're cheating with high-trigger foods like sugar and grains, you definitely run the risk of a full relapse. You'll probably find that the risk isn't worth it. Stay alert to digestive changes, and if a digestive flare-up is severe, you might want to go back to stage 1 or 2 for a few days to let things settle down again. Most people find that with the wide variety of delicious foods available, it's better to stick with full GAPS and enjoy a symptom-free life.

Milestone 2 Testing Food Intolerances

6 MONTHS INTO THE DIET By now you've determined your food allergies, sensitivities, and intolerances. After about 6 months of symptom-free eating, you might want to try to reintroduce foods you were sensitive to. You can begin by trying the Food Sensitivity Test. If you have no irritation, try a small amount of the food and wait to see if any of your symptoms return. If you're still sensitive, continue to avoid the food.

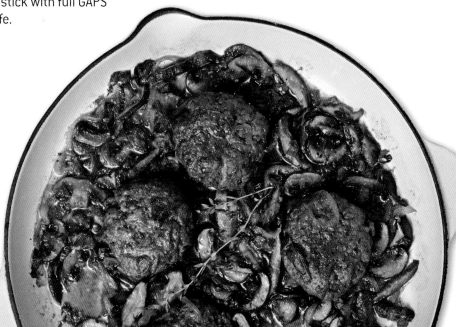

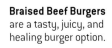
Braised Beef Burgers are a tasty, juicy, and healing burger option.

Milestone 3 Reintroducing Dairy

6 MONTHS INTO THE DIET If you had a previous dairy intolerance, you might want to try to reintroduce it after 6 months on the full GAPS diet with no digestive symptoms. Here's how:

1 Start by using ghee.

2 If you have no digestive flare-ups for 6 weeks, move on to butter.

3 If butter is tolerated, try homemade cultured cream. Start slowly, with 1 or 2 tablespoons, and build up to 1 or 2 cups per day, again waiting 6 weeks and looking for any signs of digestive distress.

4 The next step is kefir, using the same method of starting with 1 or 2 tablespoons and increasing to 1 or 2 cups per day.

5 If you tolerate kefir, you may begin with cheddar or Parmesan cheese, having a small amount with a meal and seeing how you react over the next 3 to 5 days.

6 If all goes well, you may begin to add other GAPS-legal cheeses, always using your food journal to see what effect the new foods may have on your body.

If, along this path, you react to any food, eliminate it and do not progress any further. You always can try again in 6 more months. Your gut might need more healing time, but it could be that you have a true allergy to dairy rather than an intolerance. Consult a medical professional if you suspect this is the case.

Milestone 4 Doing Another Intro

1 YEAR INTO THE DIET Many people choose to do a round of the introduction diet once or twice a year to shore up their gut lining, which can be compromised by abuse of the 80/20 rule or by other stressors. You can repeat the intro diet as often as needed, taking time off between to enjoy the full GAPS diet. Keep in mind that prolonged restricted diets can put you in danger of getting bored and frustrated and falling into binge behavior, which will make things worse rather than better.

Food Sensitivity Test

SKIN TEST

To test for a food sensitivity, follow these steps. (This test is best for liquid foods.)

1 Put a drop of the test food on the inside of your forearm before going to bed. If it's a solid food, mix it with a bit of water.

2 Leave the food overnight, and check the spot the next morning. If it's red and irritated, it's likely not tolerated.

PULSE TEST

Alternatively, you can do a pulse test. (This is handy for foods that aren't easy to skin test.)

1 Sit down, take a deep breath, and record your pulse for 1 full minute.

2 Take a bite of the food in question and chew it (but do not swallow it) for 30 seconds.

3 Take your pulse again for another full minute.

4 If your pulse has raised by 6 beats or more, the food is likely not tolerated. Spit out the food, rinse your mouth, and wait for your 1-minute pulse reading to return to normal before testing other foods.

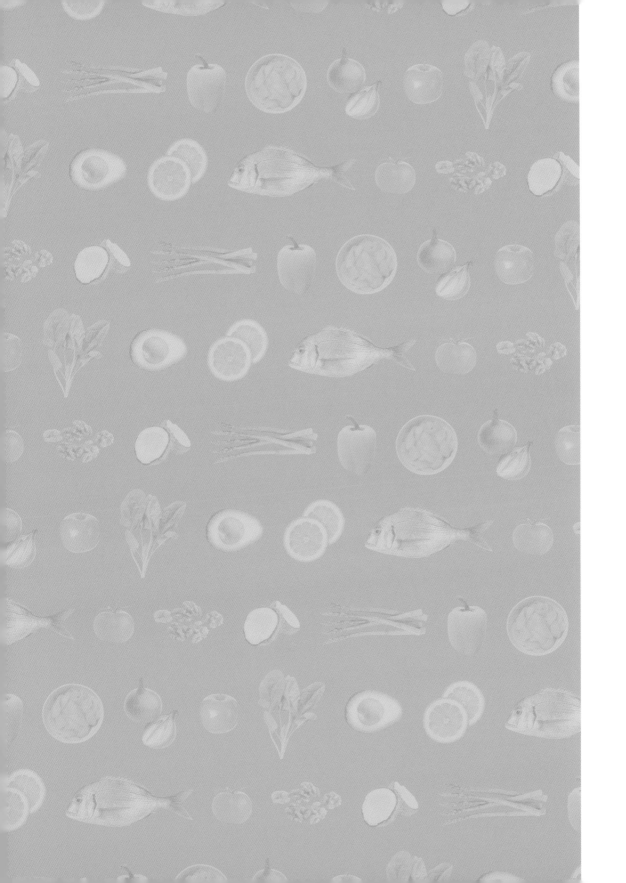

Foundation Recipes and Basics

The recipes and techniques in this part are the building blocks for the diet and its stages. Master these ferments, cultures, stocks, broths, and more, and you'll be prepared to tackle the diet with minimal stress.

DAIRY FREE

NUT FREE

PALEO DIET

Meat Stock

There's no contest between highly processed, commercially available stocks and bouillons and the homemade version. Warm and mildly meaty, homemade stock is natural and contains the minerals, vitamins, and amino acids needed to support gut health and digestion in an easy-to-process form.

Prep Time	Cook Time	Makes	Serving Size
15 minutes	3 to 5 hours	8 cups	8 cups

INGREDIENTS

5 lb (2.25kg) beef or lamb shanks

6 medium carrots, roughly chopped

6 medium stalks celery, roughly chopped

2 medium yellow onions, roughly chopped

6 cloves garlic

5 sprigs rosemary

5 sprigs thyme

3 tsp sea salt

8 whole black peppercorns

9 cups water

METHOD

1 In a large stockpot, combine beef shanks, carrots, celery, yellow onions, garlic, rosemary, thyme, sea salt, black peppercorns, and water. Set over medium-high heat, and bring to a boil.

2 Cover, reduce heat to medium-low, and simmer for 3 to 5 hours. Remove bones and meat, and set aside.

3 Strain stock through a fine-mesh strainer into a large pan and cool to 40°F (4.4°C).

4 Separate meat from bones, and refrigerate cooled meat and bones, tightly covered, for use as needed in broths and meals.

5 Refrigerate broth in heatproof jars with tight-sealing lids for up to 7 days, or freeze for up to 6 months.

DAIRY FREE **NUT FREE** **PALEO DIET**

Chicken Stock

Chicken stock makes a great base and an easy flavor-enhancer for many dishes that call for a liquid, including soups, stews, and casseroles. It's also warm, filling, and nourishing all on its own.

Prep Time
10 minutes

Cook Time
2 hours

Makes
16 cups

Serving Size
1 cups

INGREDIENTS

1 (5-lb; 2.25kg) whole roasting chicken

1 large carrot, skin on, chopped

1 large stalk celery, chopped

1 large yellow onion, skin on, chopped

1 bay leaf

10 sprigs thyme

1 tbsp black peppercorns

1 tsp sea salt

6 qt (5.5 liters) water

METHOD

1 In a large stockpot, combine chicken, carrot, celery, yellow onion, bay leaf, thyme, black peppercorns, sea salt, and water. Set over high heat, and bring to a boil.

2 Reduce heat to low, and simmer uncovered for 2 hours.

3 Remove chicken from the pot, and strain stock through a fine-mesh strainer into a large pan.

4 Pull cooked chicken from the bones, cool, and refrigerate tightly covered for future use.

5 If not using immediately, place stock pan in the sink and surround with cold water and ice cubes to cool.

6 Refrigerate in a container with a tight-sealing lid for up to 7 days, or freeze for up to 6 months.

Variations

Roasted Chicken Stock

STAGE 4

Roast the chicken first to yield a richer, deeper-flavored stock. Preheat the oven to 375°F (190°C), place chicken on a baking sheet or in a glass baking dish, and roast for 30 minutes or until skin is browned. The chicken won't be fully cooked at this point. Transfer it, and any browned bits and juices from the baking pan, to a large stockpot. Add remaining ingredients, and proceed as directed.

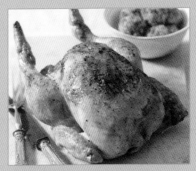

Roasted chicken is a good place to start your stock in later stages, resulting in a more flavorful dish.

Fish Stock

STAGE 1

Substitute 4 ounces (115g) fish for the chicken, and simmer for no more than 45 minutes. Use the bones, skins, fins, and heads, rather than the meat. For a lighter-flavored stock, choose mild white fish such as halibut, sole, flounder, or turbot. For a stronger stock, use salmon or bluefish.

DAIRY FREE NUT FREE PALEO DIET

Beef Bone Broth

Once you've transitioned to the full diet, you can replace stock with bone broth in your soups and for sipping between meals. Cooked over a longer time, bone broth is full of minerals and stomach-healing gelatin.

Prep Time
1 hour, 15 minutes

Cook Time
24 to 72 hours

Makes
4 quarts (4 liters)

Serving Size
1 cup

INGREDIENTS

4 qt (4 liters) spring or filtered water

½ cup apple cider vinegar

1 (3- or 4-lb; 1.5–2kg) beef knuckle and marrow bones

2 lb (1kg) meaty bones such as oxtail or short ribs

2 medium stalks celery, chopped into thirds

2 large carrots, peeled and coarsely chopped

2 medium yellow onions, cut into quarters

Unrefined sea salt (no additives)

METHOD

1 In a large stockpot, combine spring water, apple cider vinegar, beef knuckle and marrow bones, and meaty bones, adding more water to completely cover bones if needed.

2 Add celery, carrots, and yellow onions. Set heat to high, and bring to a boil, skimming any scum off top as needed.

3 Reduce heat to medium-low, cover, and simmer for 24 to 72 hours. (You can use a slow cooker for this if you like.) The longer broth simmers, the more gelatin is released.

4 Strain broth through a fine-mesh strainer. Return any bone marrow to broth, and season with sea salt. Cool to 40°F (4.4°C).

5 Refrigerate broth in heatproof jars with tight-sealing lids for up to 7 days, or freeze for up to 6 months.

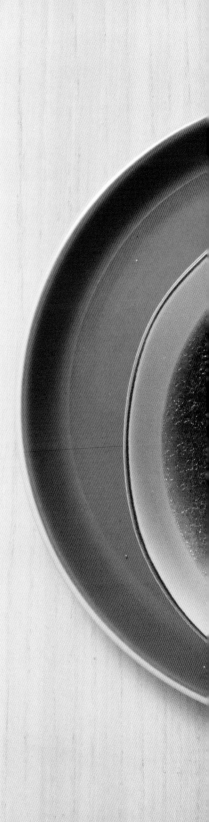

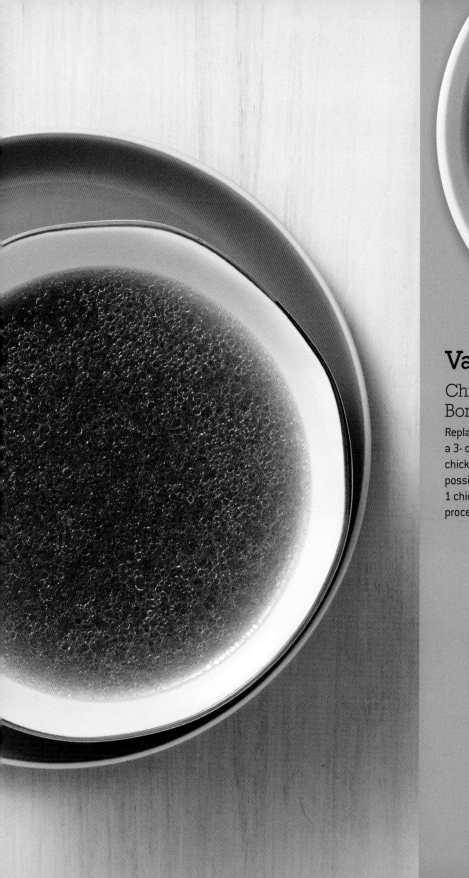

Variation

Chicken Bone Broth

FULL DIET

Replace beef bones with a 3- or 4-pound (1.5–2kg) chicken, organic and pastured if possible; 2 to 4 chicken feet; and 1 chicken neck (optional). Then proceed as directed.

Fermenting Basics

Fermented or cultured vegetables are an integral part of the gut-healing process because they repopulate the gut with beneficial bacteria, which help restore balance to your microbiome. Any vegetable can be fermented.

Choose Organic

Choose organic vegetables if possible. Fermenting increases the vitamin and mineral content of the vegetables so it's best to start with vegetables at the peak of freshness.

- Cabbage is the most popular vegetable used for fermentation.
- Turnips and other root vegetables ferment well.
- Vegetables such as peppers or carrots can be added for color and flavor. Experiment to find out what you like!

Sterilize Your Equipment

It's essential all your jars and utensils are clean before fermenting. You're creating a bacteria-friendly environment, so it's important no undesirable bacteria remain that could multiply.

- Pulling jars directly out of the dishwasher after the drying cycle ensures sterility.
- If you suspect cleanliness issues, submerge your jars and utensils in boiling water to sterilize them.
- It's more likely the good bacteria would crowd out any bad bacteria, but it's better to be safe than sorry.

Simple Sauerkraut

You can use these steps to ferment other vegetables as well.

INGREDIENTS

1 medium head
cabbage
1 tbsp sea salt
Spring or filtered
water

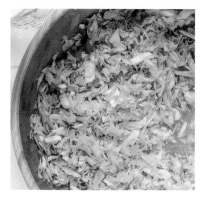

1 Remove the outer 2 or 3 leaves from head of cabbage, and thinly slice cabbage using a chef's knife.

2 Place sliced cabbage in a large bowl. With clean hands, begin to work cabbage, squeezing and massaging it until it starts to release liquid. (This is called the brine.)

Culturing Tips

Keep these tips in mind when you're culturing vegetables.

- Vegetables culture at room temperature, so find a place in your kitchen or home where they can sit out of direct sunlight for at least 7 days.

- For a more sour taste, ferment until your desired taste, testing every week. When they reach your desired flavor, refrigerate to slow fermentation.

- The more sour the taste, the more beneficial bacteria is present. You might find that your taste buds change and your body begins to crave these friendly microbes.

- Glass jars and lids are easy to find online or at your local discount or hardware store.

- Be sure you have large bowls to accommodate the vegetables as you shred and mix them.

- You can use a spatula or spoon to pack the vegetables into the jars. No need for fancy equipment!

NO FERMENTED FRUIT

You can ferment fruits as well as vegetables, although more care must be taken when working with fruits because the sugar in them produces small amounts of alcohol when fermented. Fermented fruit is not appropriate for a gut-healing protocol.

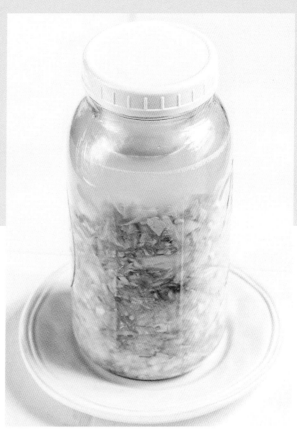

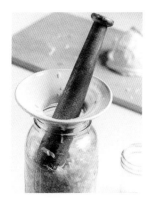

3 Tightly pack shredded cabbage into 1-quart (1-liter) glass jars. Use your hands, a spatula, or any sturdy kitchen tool to press firmly. Add sea salt.

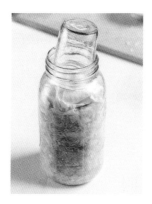

4 Use a small glass to pack down cabbage one last time, leaving 2 inches (5cm) breathing space at the top of the jar. Add the lid, close firmly, and then loosen a quarter turn.

5 If cabbage has not produced enough brine on its own, fill the jar with water until cabbage is completely submerged. Let the jars sit at room temperature out of direct sunlight for 7 days. "Burp" the jars each day by opening the lids, closing firmly, and then loosening a quarter turn. Taste sauerkraut after 7 days. For a more sour flavor, ferment for up to 2 weeks. Store in the refrigerator for up to 6 months.

DAIRY FREE **LOW FODMAP**

Red Cabbage Kraut

Crisp and tangy, this colorful, purple, 7-day ferment is rich in probiotics, vitamins, and minerals that support gut health. Use the juice in stages 1 and 2 and the kraut in stage 3.

Prep Time	Cook Time	Makes	Serving Size
20 minutes	7 days	2 (1-quart; 1-liter) jars	¼ cup

INGREDIENTS

¼ cup unrefined sea salt (no additives)

8 cups filtered, unchlorinated mineral water

1 medium head red cabbage, stemmed, cored, and shredded thin

METHOD

1 In a medium bowl, dissolve sea salt in mineral water.

2 Pack red cabbage tightly into 1-quart (1-liter) glass jars. Pour brine into jars over cabbage, packing down cabbage so it's completely submerged, and leaving at least 1 or 2 inches (2.5cm or 5cm) head space at the top of the jar.

3 Cover the jars with the lids, and set aside at room temperature out of direct sunlight for 7 days.

4 Once daily, loosen the lids to allow gasses to escape. Press down on cabbage as needed to ensure it remains submerged in brine. Retighten the lids.

5 Refrigerate for up to 6 months.

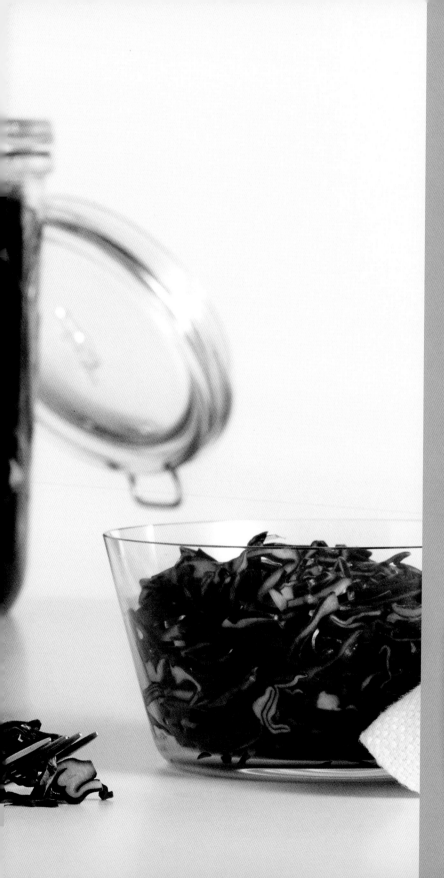

Variation

Sweet-and-Sour Red Slaw

STAGE 6

Combine $1/2$ cup Red Cabbage Kraut; $1/2$ cup crisp sliced red apple; $1/4$ cup shredded carrot; 1 tablespoon unsweetened, unsulfured raisins; 1 tablespoon walnuts; and 1 tablespoon virgin olive oil.

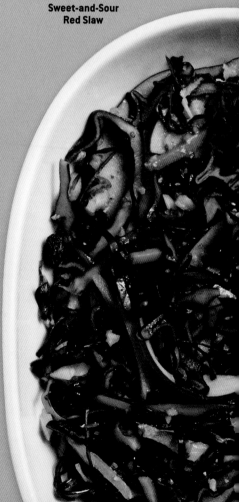

Sweet-and-Sour Red Slaw

DAIRY FREE

NUT FREE

PALEO DIET

Fermented Mixed Vegetables

In this gut-healing giardiniera, bright-colored, mild-flavored, textured vegetables make a great standalone snack or a perfect condiment for meats, fish, or eggs. Incorporate the juice starting in stage 1, and add the vegetables when you get to stage 3.

Prep Time	Cook Time	Makes	Serving Size
15 minutes	6 days	4 cups	$^1/_2$ cup

INGREDIENTS

- 2 tbsp unrefined sea salt (no additives)
- 4 cups filtered, unchlorinated, mineral water
- 1 cup carrot, peeled and cut into $^1/_2$-in (1.25cm) rounds
- 1 cup yellow bell pepper, ribs and seeds removed, and cut into 1-in (2.5cm) squares
- 1 cup red bell pepper, ribs and seeds removed, and cut into 1-in (2.5cm) squares
- 1 cup cauliflower florets, cut into 1-in (2.5cm) pieces
- 4 cloves garlic, halved

METHOD

1 In a small bowl, dissolve sea salt in water.

2 Using a wooden spoon, tightly pack carrot, yellow bell pepper, red bell pepper, cauliflower, and garlic into a 1-quart (1-liter) glass jar. Add water, leaving 1 or 2 inches (2.5 to 5cm) headspace at the top of the jar. Press down vegetables, if necessary, to completely submerge.

3 Cover the jar with the lid, and set aside at room temperature out of direct sunlight for 6 days.

4 Once daily, loosen the lid to allow gasses to escape. Press down on vegetables as needed to ensure they remain submerged. Retighten the lid.

5 Refrigerate for up to 6 months.

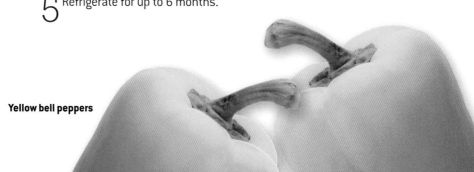

Yellow bell peppers

STAGE 4

DAIRY FREE

NUT FREE

PALEO DIET

Cultured Spring Vegetables

Colorful, flavorful, probiotic-rich cultured vegetables help rebalance gut flora. Start with small amounts of juice in stages 1 and 2, and slowly build up to 2 to 4 tablespoons vegetables with each meal in stage 3.

Prep Time
20 minutes

Cook Time
6 days

Makes
4 (1-quart; 1-liter) jars

Serving Size
¼ cup

INGREDIENTS

1 medium head green cabbage

1 medium yellow squash

1 medium zucchini

2 large carrots

4 cups thinly sliced kale

4 tsp sea salt

Spring or filtered water

METHOD

1 In a food processor fitted with a metal chopping blade, shred green cabbage, yellow squash, zucchini, and carrots.

2 Transfer shredded vegetables to a large bowl, add kale, and stir to combine.

3 Pack vegetables into 1-quart (1-liter) glass jars, pressing firmly with a spatula. Leave 2 or 3 inches (5 to 7.5cm) at the top of the jar.

4 Add 1 teaspoon sea salt to each jar, and fill with water, completely submerging vegetables. Seal jars tightly with lids.

5 Let jars sit at room temperature out of direct sunlight for 6 days.

6 Store in refrigerator for up to 6 months.

Variations

Cultured Root Vegetables

STAGE 4

Replace the yellow squash with 1 medium beet, and instead of the zucchini, use 1 medium turnip. Decrease the kale to 2 cups, and add 1 cup radishes. Shred beet, turnip, and radishes, and combine with the other vegetables as directed.

Cultured Rainbow Vegetables

STAGE 4

Use red cabbage. Replace the yellow squash with 2 yellow bell peppers, ribs and seeds removed, and instead of the zucchini, use 2 orange bell peppers, ribs and seeds removed. Decrease the kale to 2 cups, and add 2 red bell peppers, ribs and seeds removed. Shred the bell peppers, and combine with the other vegetables as directed.

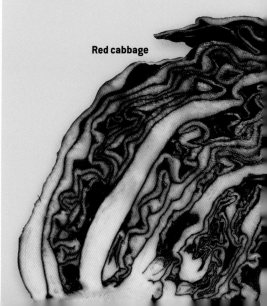

Red cabbage

**LOW
FODMAP**

**NUT
FREE**

Home-Churned Butter

It's hard to beat the creamy texture and rich flavor of fresh, homemade butter—so silky smooth, you'll never choose store-bought butter again. This easy recipe provides a quality foundation for homemade ghee as well.

Prep Time
15 minutes

Makes
1 pound (450g)

Serving Size
1 tablespoon

INGREDIENTS

4 cups organic, grass-fed, raw heavy cream, or organic, lightly pasteurized, nonhomogenized heavy cream

METHOD

1 Using a food processor fitted with a metal blade, a blender, or a stand mixer fitted with metal whisk attachment, whip heavy cream on low speed. Increase speed to medium as cream starts to thicken.

2 When cream has solidified into butter and liquid forms in the bowl, stop whipping. Discard liquid in the bowl.

3 Transfer butter to the middle of a piece of cheesecloth large enough to wrap butter completely. Wash cheesecloth-wrapped butter under cold water, squeezing butter as you rinse, until water runs clear.

4 Pack butter into an airtight container, or wrap in plastic wrap, and refrigerate for several weeks or freeze for up to 9 months.

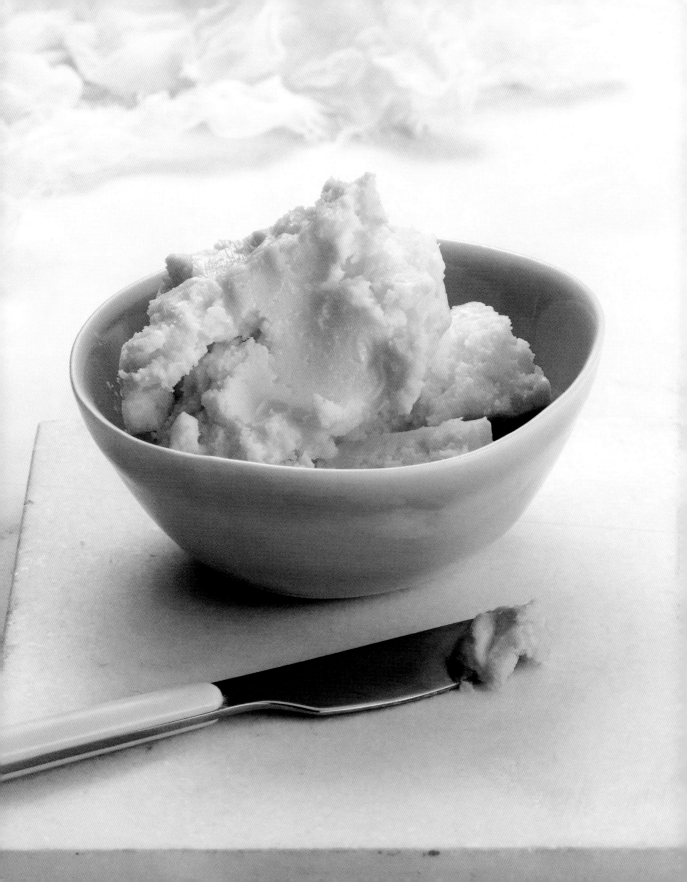

NUT FREE

LOW FODMAP

Ghee

Ghee has a rich, nutty taste and minimal milk solids and lactose. Use it as you would butter. It's also good to add to soups and broths for extra gut-healing fat.

Prep Time	Cook Time	Makes	Serving Size
2 minutes	20 to 30 minutes	2 scant cups	1 tablespoon

INGREDIENTS

1 lb (450g) unsalted butter

METHOD

1 In a medium saucepan over medium heat, melt unsalted butter for 10 to 15 minutes.

2 As butter begins to bubble, reduce heat to medium-low. Skim off foam as it develops, and cook, allowing browned milk solids to form and drop to the bottom of the pan, for 10 to 15 more minutes.

3 Strain ghee through a fine-mesh strainer lined with cheesecloth into an airtight, heatproof container.

4 Store at room temperature for up to 6 months.

Ghee

> You also can cook the butter in a slow cooker on low for 6 to 8 hours. Skim off the foam if desired, or allow it to sink to the bottom. Strain as directed.

STAGE 4

DAIRY FREE

PALEO DIET

Nut Milk

If you can't tolerate dairy, nut milk is an excellent alternative. And by making it yourself, you can avoid unwanted sugars and chemicals and maximize your nutrient absorption.

Prep Time
15 minutes

Makes
3 or 4 cups

Serving Size
1 cup milk

INGREDIENTS

- 1 cup nuts, soaked overnight
- 4 cups very hot spring or filtered water

METHOD

1 In a high-speed blender, blend nuts and hot spring water for 2 minutes.

2 Transfer mixture to a nut milk bag or a fine-mesh strainer lined with cheesecloth, and gently squeeze bag or press down on solids to strain milk into the bowl. Thin milk with more spring water if needed to achieve your desired consistency.

3 Refrigerate in a glass jar for up to 3 days.

Variations

Coconut Milk

STAGE 6

Use 5 cups very hot spring or filtered water, and swap out the nuts for 3 cups unsweetened coconut flakes. Blend for 3 minutes, and proceed as directed.

Flavored Nut Milk

FULL DIET

When you reach the full diet stage, you can make your nut milk a little more interesting by adding spices or sweeteners. Try adding cinnamon, nutmeg, or honey after step 2.

Coconut

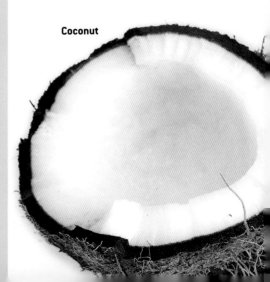

Cultured Dairy Basics

Cultured dairy helps repopulate your gut with beneficial bacteria that restore balance to your microbiome. Milk and cream can be cultured in a variety of ways for different tastes and results.

THE IMPORTANCE OF STERILIZATION

Dairy should be cultured in clean, dry glass jars so there are no opportunistic bacteria that might spoil the culture. Using jars fresh out of the dishwasher is ideal. You can sterilize jars in boiling water for 30 to 60 seconds if you suspect they may be contaminated. Be sure your utensils also are clean and dry.

Kefir

Kefir is a sour-tasting drink made of cow's or goat's milk.

- Kefir has the highest number of beneficial bacteria and yeast among cultured dairy products.

- It contains kefirans, which have shown potential as anticancer agents in scientific research.

- Homemade kefir includes the full complement of bacteria and yeast store-bought lacks.

Cultured Dairy

Cultured dairy is simple to make, although you might need to make adjustments based on the temperature in your kitchen. It'll be worth it!

INGREDIENTS

4 cups organic, grass-fed raw or lightly pasteurized/ vat pasteurized nonhomogenized whole milk

1/4 cup organic commercial yogurt or powdered starter

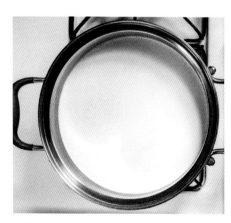

1 Heat dairy to about 90°F (32°C) to activate cultures. If you're using raw milk, you can scald it by heating it to 180°F (82°C) to kill any native beneficial bacteria that can change the flavor. If you do scald, don't add starter until the milk's temperature drops to 90°F (32°C).

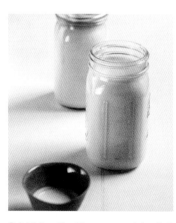

2 Add 1 or 2 tablespoons of the finished product to heated milk, or use a dried starter culture. (The first time you use a dried starter, you might need additional time for culturing because the culture is waking up after having been dried. Jars should be clean and dry.)

Yogurt

Yogurt, the most familiar cultured dairy, is slightly thicker than kefir and easy to make.

- By law, yogurt must contain *Lactobacillus bulgaricus* and *Streptococcus thermophilus.*

- There are two types of yogurt starter: thermophilic, or heat-loving, starter and mesophilic starter, which does not need to be heated.

- Homemade yogurt won't be as thick as commercially made yogurt. To thicken, you can to strain it through layers of cheesecloth in a strainer set over a bowl. Pour in the yogurt, and allow it to sit for several hours or until it reaches your desired consistency.

Cultured Cream and Butter

Cultured cream and butter are healthy condiments that provide both flavor and nutrients.

- The higher the fat content of the cream, the thicker your cultured cream will be. If you want thicker cultured cream, scald the cream and let it cool for 30 minutes before culturing.

- Butter made with milk from cows who have grazed on grass has a rich, golden color that indicates its high nutrient content.

- Both cream and butter are excellent sources of vitamins A, D, E, and K as well as cholesterol, which is the building block of every cell in your body.

BUYING DAIRY FOR CULTURING

You can make cultured dairy with raw milk or pasteurized milk. Raw milk has many health benefits. The natural bacteria in milk may slightly alter the taste of the finished product as they interact with the culture that's been added. If you're buying pasteurized milk, try to get milk that's been lightly pasteurized or vat pasteurized. Avoid ultrapasteurized (UHT) milk. The proteins in this type of milk have been denatured and, therefore, have lost much of their vitality. Avoid homogenized milk, too; its fats are difficult to assimilate.

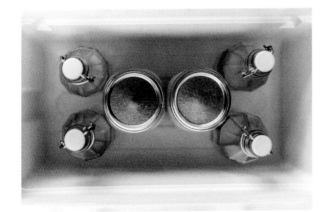

3 Allow dairy to cool to room temperature. Then, let dairy cultures sit at room temperature, out of direct sunlight, for 24 hours. The temperature of your kitchen has a big impact on the culturing time. If your kitchen is cool, you can culture your jars in a cooler.

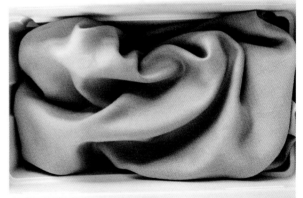

4 Cover the jars in the cooler with a blanket or towel to maintain the right temperature. If your dairy separates before 24 hours, you might need less time due to a warmer kitchen, or you might have used too much starter.

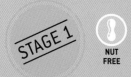

STAGE 1

NUT
FREE

Yogurt

Tangy, silky yogurt is easy to make and much healthier than store-bought versions. In later stages of the protocol, you can add properly soaked and dried nuts or unsweetened, flaked coconut and season with cinnamon, nutmeg, and organic vanilla extract.

Prep Time	**Cook Time**	**Makes**	**Serving Size**
2 minutes	24 hours	4 cups	½ cup

INGREDIENTS

- 4 cups organic, grass-fed, raw, or lightly pasteurized/vat pasteurized nonhomogenized whole milk
- ¼ cup organic commercial yogurt

METHOD

1 In a medium saucepan over low heat, heat milk for about 10 minutes or until it reaches 180°F (80°C). (Use a thermometer.) If you're using raw milk, heat it to 110°F (40°C).

2 Remove from heat, and allow milk to cool for about 10 minutes or until it reaches 110°F (40°C).

3 Place yogurt in a 1-quart (1-liter) glass jar with a tight-fitting lid, and fill jar with warm milk, leaving 1 inch (2.5cm) at the top.

4 Place jar in a yogurt maker or a dehydrator set to 110°F (40°C) or in oven with the light on for 24 hours.

5 Allow yogurt to cool in the refrigerator.

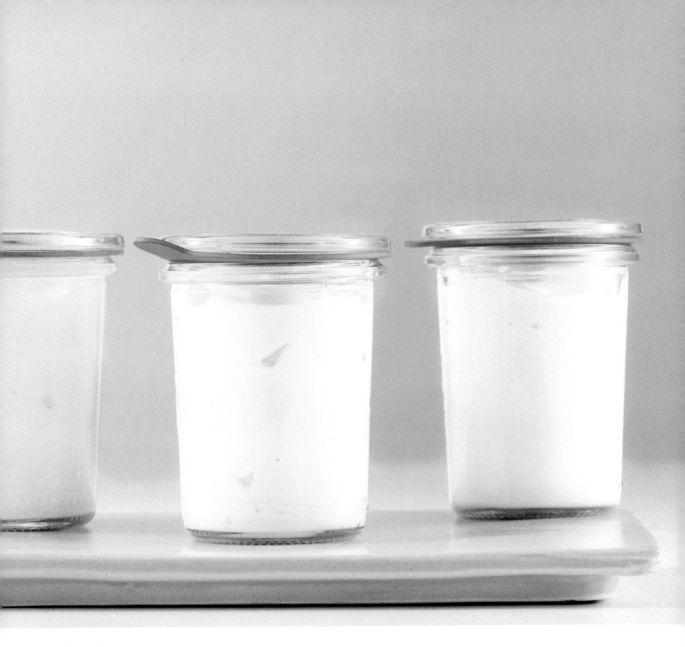

Variations

Coconut Milk Yogurt

STAGE 6

Substitute 1 (13.5-ounce; 383g) can full-fat coconut milk for the organic whole milk. Shake the can vigorously before opening. Add 1 probiotic capsule to the coconut milk, and culture as directed.

Almond Milk Yogurt

STAGE 4

Substitute 4 cups almond milk for the organic whole milk. After heating the milk, add 1 tablespoon raw honey and 1 or 2 probiotic capsules. Culture milk as directed.

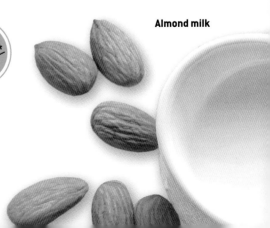

Almond milk

NUT
FREE

Cultured Cream

Cultured cream, or what many people think of as sour cream, is an excellent addition to soups if you can tolerate dairy. If you've been choosing low-fat sour cream, this rich food might feel like you're cheating.

Prep Time	Cook Time	Makes	Serving Size
5 minutes	24 to 48 hours	4 cups	2 tablespoons

INGREDIENTS

4 cups organic, grass-fed raw, or lightly pasteurized/vat pasteurized nonhomogenized cream

$^1/_4$ cup homemade yogurt, previously made cultured cream, or yogurt starter

METHOD

1 In a large saucepan over medium heat, heat cream to 185°F (85°C), and hold it at that temperature for 45 minutes, watching the temperature carefully.

2 Remove from heat, and cool cream to 77°F (25°C).

3 Pour cooled cream into a glass jar with a tight-fitting lid. Add homemade yogurt.

4 Seal the jar, and set aside out of direct sunlight for 24 hours. If your kitchen is cooler than 74°F (23°C), place jars in a cooler with the lid closed while culturing.

5 Check cream for consistency. If it's not thickened enough, set aside for up to 48 hours.

Variations

Cultured Butter

Follow the Cultured Cream instructions. After the cream has cultured, refrigerate it until the cream is cooled to 60°F (15.5°C). Proceed as directed in the Home-Churned Butter recipe.

STAGE 1

Crème Fraîche

Use $^1/_4$ cup store-bought cultured buttermilk instead of yogurt, previously made cultured cream, or yogurt starter.

STAGE 1

**NUT
FREE**

Kefir

Kefir is a powerhouse of probiotics. Given its tart taste, you might want to sweeten it with honey. Whatever your preference, your gut will thank you for making it a regular part of your diet.

Prep Time	**Cook Time**	**Makes**	**Serving Size**
5 minutes	24 hours	4 cups	¹/₂ cup

INGREDIENTS

- 4 cups organic, grass-fed raw or lightly pasteurized/vat pasteurized and nonhomogenized whole milk
- 1 packet kefir starter or 2 tbsp kefir grains

METHOD

1 In a medium saucepan over medium heat, heat milk to 180°F (82°C). (Use a thermometer.) If you're using raw milk, heat to 110°F (40°C).

2 Cool milk to 110°F (40°C) (if necessary, place the pot in the sink and surround with cold water and ice cubes to cool milk quickly), and pour into a 1-quart (1-liter) glass jar along with kefir starter.

3 Seal the jar and set aside at room temperature out of direct sunlight for 24 hours. Occasionally shake the jar to ensure all milk is fermenting.

4 Strain kefir into a fresh jar, and use grains to start another batch. If using starter, reserve ¹/₂ cup kefir to start the next batch.

Variations

Coconut Milk Kefir

Substitute 4 cups coconut milk for the whole milk if you can't tolerate dairy. Do not heat the coconut milk. Proceed as described.

Flavored Kefir

Use a second fermentation. Add ¹/₄ cup of your favorite fruit to the jar, cap tightly, and let ferment at room temperature for another 24 hours.

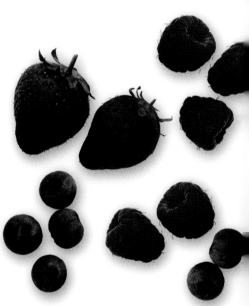

Fresh berries

**DAIRY
FREE**

**PALEO
DIET**

Everyday Grain-Free Bread

You'll be glad zero grain doesn't mean zero bread after tasting a slice of this loaf, which provides a soft, warm, nutty experience you'll love. Because this bread is so nourishing, it's no problem reaching for a second slice, especially with a spread of homemade butter.

Prep Time	Cook Time	Makes	Serving Size
15 minutes	40 minutes	1 loaf/14 slices	1 slice

INGREDIENTS

6 large eggs

$^1/_4$ cup coconut oil

$^1/_2$ tsp apple cider vinegar

$^3/_4$ cup smooth almond butter

2 tbsp raw honey

$^1/_4$ cup hazelnut flour/meal

$^1/_4$ cup homemade coconut flour

1 tsp baking soda

$^3/_4$ tsp sea salt

METHOD

1 Preheat the oven to 350°F (180°C). Line a $8^1/_2 \times 4^1/_2$-inch (21.6×11.4cm) loaf pan with parchment paper so the paper extends over all sides of the pan by 2 inches (5cm).

2 In a medium bowl, whisk together eggs, coconut oil, apple cider vinegar, almond butter, and honey.

3 In a separate medium bowl, combine hazelnut flour, coconut flour, baking soda, and sea salt.

4 Slowly mix dry ingredients into wet ingredients until well combined, and transfer dough to the prepared loaf pan.

5 Bake on the middle oven rack for 45 minutes.

6 Remove the pan from the oven, and allow to cool completely. To remove bread from the pan, lift the edges of the parchment paper.

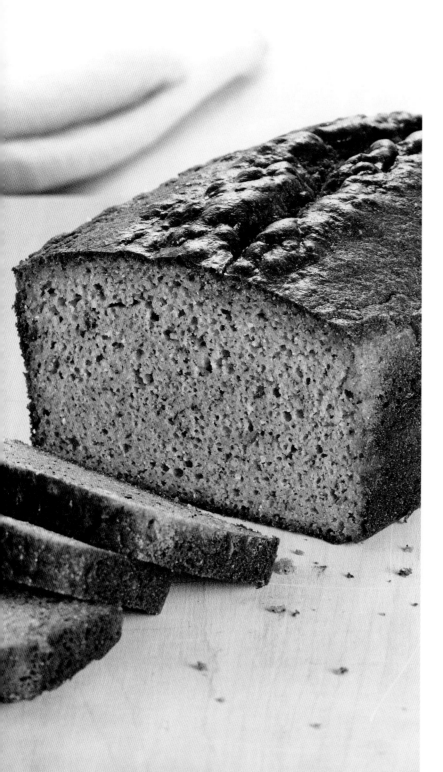

Component

Homemade Coconut Flour

STAGE 4

Homemade coconut flour is lighter, fluffier, and much lower in fiber than commercial versions. Here's how to make your own.

INGREDIENTS
1 Thai coconut
2½ cups filtered water

METHOD

1 Remove the thick husk from Thai coconut until rounded top is visible. Using a heavy knife, make 4 marks against the top, creating a 2-inch (5cm) square. Continue to strike the four marks until coconut opens. Drain out coconut water.

2 Using a spoon, scrape coconut meat from inside shell, and place in a small bowl. Using a ratio of 1 cup meat to 2½ cups filtered water, place meat and water in a blender, and blend for 1 minute or until smooth. Strain blended coconut through a cheesecloth or fine-mesh strainer, reserving coconut milk for another use.

3 Preheat the oven to 100°F (38°C). Spread strained coconut pulp on a baking sheet lined with parchment paper, and bake for 1 hour or until moisture has evaporated and pulp is dried. Allow coconut to cool.

4 Process cooled, dried coconut pulp in a blender for 30 seconds or until it's a fine powder. Refrigerate tightly covered until ready to use.

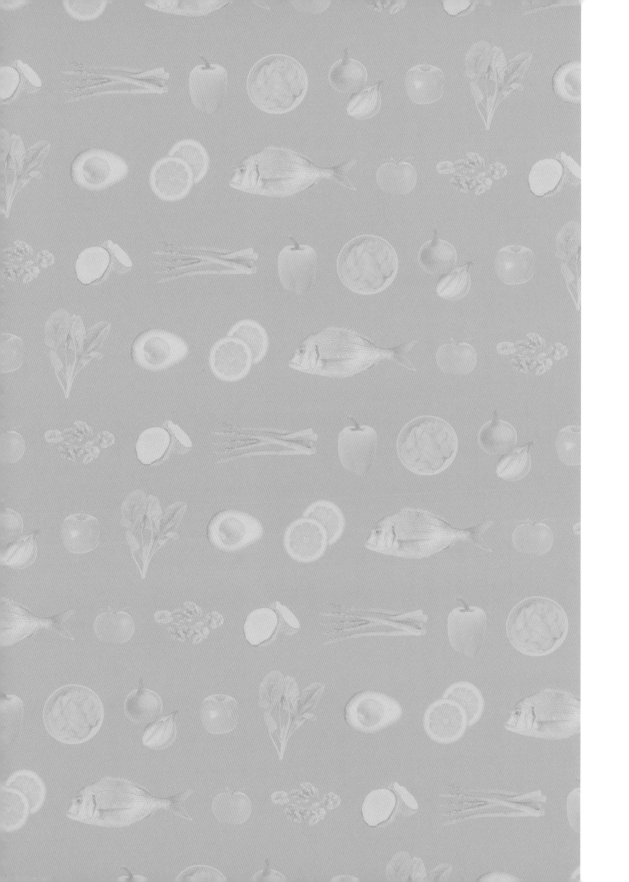

Recipes by Stage

This part contains more than 150 recipes that progress through the diet. From soups to entrées, sides, salads, breakfasts, snacks, desserts, and more, these delicious recipes soothe your gut and provide a variety of flavors and textures.

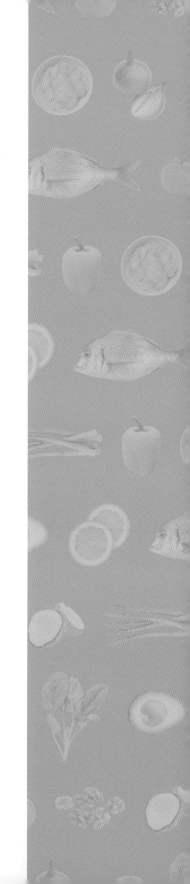

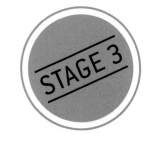

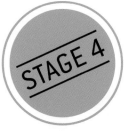

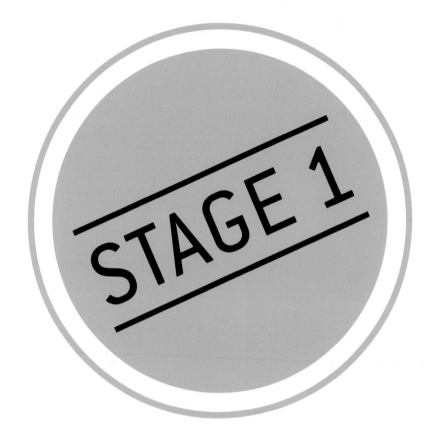

STAGE 1

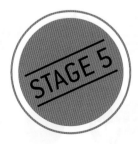

STAGE 5

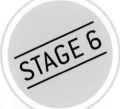

STAGE 6

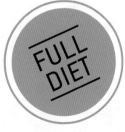

FULL
DIET

DAIRY FREE **NUT FREE** **PALEO DIET**

Classic Chicken Soup

This classic soup will likely become a go-to meal in stages 1 and 2. It's quick, easy, tasty, and very good for your gut. Don't forget to add the fat for the extra gut-healing boost.

Prep Time
20 minutes

Cook Time
20 minutes

Makes
8 to 10 cups

Serving Size
1 cup

INGREDIENTS

- 8 cups homemade chicken stock
- 2 medium carrots, peeled and cut into ¼-in (0.5cm) slices
- 2 large stalks celery, cut into ¼-in (0.5cm) slices
- 1 medium yellow onion, sliced medium
- 2 tsp sea salt
- 3 or 4 black peppercorns
- 1 or 2 cups cooked, shredded chicken reserved from making stock (optional)
- 2 tbsp animal fat or coconut oil

METHOD

1 In a large stockpot over high heat, bring chicken stock to a boil.

2 Reduce heat to medium-low, and add carrots, celery, yellow onion, sea salt, black peppercorns, and chicken (if using). Simmer for 20 minutes. (For earlier stages, you might want to put the peppercorns in a bouquet garni bag or tie them in cheesecloth for easier removal. In stage 3, you can add 1 tablespoon finely chopped fresh parsley in the last 5 minutes of cooking. After stage 4, you can add ½ teaspoon dried basil.)

3 Serve immediately with 1 or 2 teaspoons animal fat in each bowl.

Variation

Lemon Chicken "Rice" Soup

STAGE 1

METHOD

1 Replace all the vegetables with ½ head of cauliflower florets, very finely diced into rice size with a knife or a food processor fitted with a metal chopping blade.

2 After bringing the stock to a boil, reduce heat to medium-low, add cauliflower, and cook for 10 minutes. Remove from heat, and add the juice of 2 small lemons.

3 In a medium bowl, beat 3 egg whites until they form stiff peaks. Fold in 3 beaten egg yolks, and add to the soup by spoonfuls, mixing well after each. Soup will foam and develop a thicker body. Serve immediately.

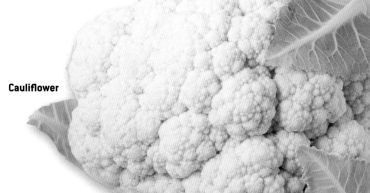

Cauliflower

DAIRY FREE   NUT FREE   PALEO DIET

Butternut Squash Soup

This warming soup is the perfect comfort food to carry you through the first two stages of the GAPS protocol. In later stages, you can add cinnamon, nutmeg, and orange zest.

Prep Time
15 minutes

Cook Time
20 minutes

Makes
10 to 12 cups

Serving Size
1½ cups

Variation

Chunky Butternut Kale Soup

STAGE 1

Use 1 medium peeled, seeded, and diced butternut squash; 1 cup diced yellow onion; 2 cloves peeled and sliced garlic; 2 medium peeled and diced carrots; 4 cups trimmed, cut kale leaves; 1 tablespoon sea salt; and 2 quarts (2 liters) homemade chicken stock. Proceed as directed in step 2.

INGREDIENTS

- 1 medium butternut squash, peeled, split, seeded, and cut into 1-in (2.5cm) dice
- 1 medium sweet or yellow onion, chopped
- 2 qt (2 liters) homemade chicken stock
- 1 tbsp sea salt
- 2 or 3 tbsp coconut oil, lard, butter, or ghee

METHOD

1 In a large stockpot, combine butternut squash, sweet onion, chicken stock, and sea salt. Set over high heat, and bring to a boil.

2 Reduce heat to medium-low, and simmer for 20 minutes or until squash has softened.

3 Working in small batches, blend soup in a blender until smooth. Return soup to the pot, and simmer for 5 more minutes or until soup has reached desired thickness.

4 To serve, add 2 or 3 teaspoons coconut oil to each bowl, and ladle hot soup over to melt.

CUTTING BUTTERNUT SQUASH

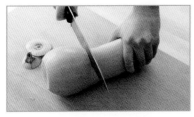

1 Cut off the top and bottom of the squash, and cut squash in half.

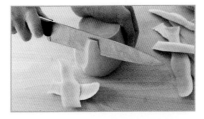

2 Remove the skin using a sharp knife or a vegetable peeler.

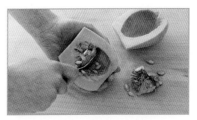

3 Scoop out the seeds with a spoon, and dice squash.

DAIRY FREE

NUT FREE

PALEO DIET

Carrot Beet Soup

Beets aid in the production of healthy bile, which helps you digest all the gut-healing fats you're adding to your diet. This richly colored soup also is full of antioxidants and phytonutrients—but you won't be thinking about that when you taste its subtle sweetness.

Prep Time	Cook Time	Makes	Serving Size
20 minutes	30 minutes	12 to 14 cups	1 cups

INGREDIENTS

- 8 cups homemade beef or chicken stock
- 6 small or 4 medium beets, peeled and quartered
- 4 medium carrots, peeled and cut in thirds
- 1 medium sweet or yellow onion, roughly chopped
- 2 cloves garlic, crushed
- 6 to 8 tbsp animal fat or coconut oil
- 1 tbsp sea salt

METHOD

1. In a large stockpot, combine beef stock, beets, carrots, sweet onion, garlic, and 2 or 3 tablespoons animal fat. Set over medium-high heat, and bring to a boil.

2. Add sea salt, lower heat to medium-low, and simmer for 20 minutes.

3. Working in small batches, blend soup in a blender until smooth. (Or use a hand blender.) If you want a thicker soup, simmer again for up to 10 more minutes.

4. Ladle into bowls, add 1 or 2 teaspoons remaining animal fat to each portion, and serve.

Occasionally, the blended carrot will begin to separate from the soup and form a bright-orange foam. This is normal; just stir it back together.

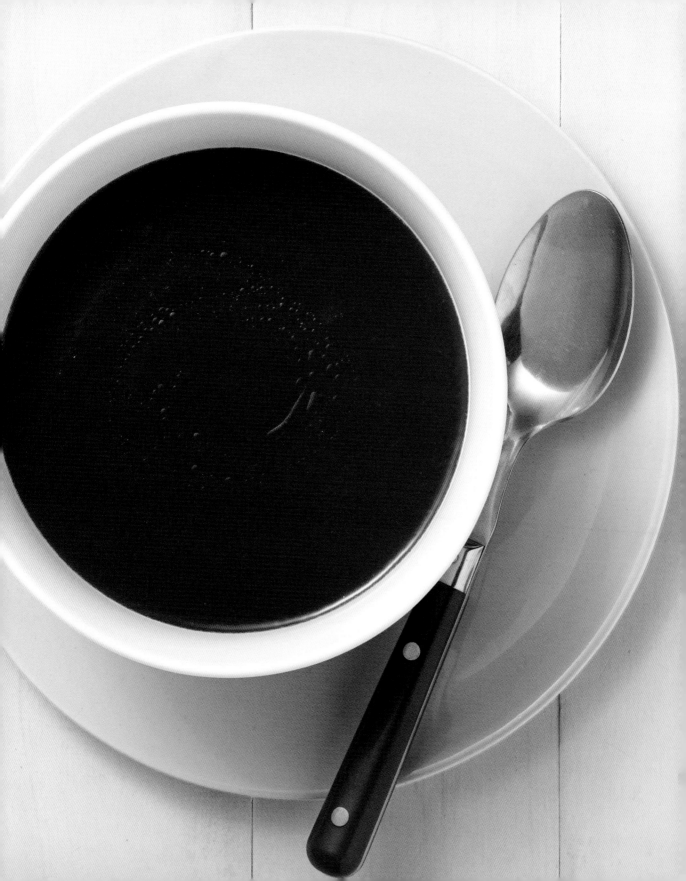

DAIRY FREE

NUT FREE

PALEO DIET

Chicken Vegetable Soup

When it comes to vegetables, more is better, and this warm, hearty, colorful intro soup is packed with them. It's also a great dish for using tender shredded stock chicken.

Prep Time	Cook Time	Makes	Serving Size
15 minutes	25 minutes	8 cups	2 cups

INGREDIENTS

4 cups homemade chicken stock

2 cups cooked shredded chicken (from stock or leftover poached)

$^3/_4$ cup carrots, peeled and cut into $^1/_2$-in (1.25cm) pieces

$^3/_4$ cup red onion, diced into $^1/_2$-in (1.25cm) pieces

4 cloves garlic, sliced thin

$^1/_2$ cup yellow bell pepper, ribs and seeds removed, and cut into $^1/_2$-in (1.25cm) pieces

$^3/_4$ cup broccoli, stem removed and cut into $^1/_2$-in (1.25cm) florets

$^3/_4$ cup cauliflower, stem and core removed and cut into $^1/_2$-in (1.25cm) florets

2 cups tomatoes, cored and diced into $^1/_2$-in (1.25cm) pieces

1 tbsp sea salt

METHOD

1 In a medium stockpot, combine chicken stock, chicken, carrots, red onion, garlic, yellow bell pepper, broccoli, cauliflower, tomatoes, and sea salt. Set over medium-high heat, and bring to a boil.

2 Reduce heat to medium-low, and simmer for 25 minutes or until vegetables are tender.

3 If not serving immediately, place the pot in the sink and surround with cold water and ice cubes to cool soup quickly.

4 Refrigerate tightly covered for 1 week, or freeze for up to 6 months.

Q&A

How do I freeze extra soup?

Doubling or tripling a soup recipe can save you time and effort later if you freeze some of the extra soup in individual portions. To freeze soup, be sure it's completely cool before freezing. Place cooled soup in containers or zipper-lock plastic freezer bags, leaving about 1 or 2 inches (2.5–5cm) headroom at the top to allow for expansion. Label and date the container, and freeze for up to 6 months.

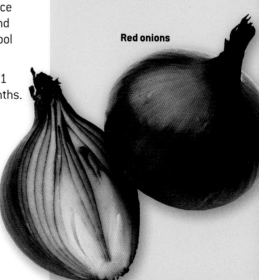
Red onions

DAIRY FREE

NUT FREE

PALEO DIET

Garlicky Greens Soup

The slight bitterness of dark, leafy greens balances the sweetness of cooked garlic in this soup. If fresh greens aren't available, use frozen, thawed spinach instead.

Prep Time
10 minutes

Cook Time
15 minutes

Makes
8 cups

Serving Size
2 cups

INGREDIENTS

- 2 cups roughly chopped baby spinach
- 2 cups chopped Swiss chard leaves, tough stem removed
- 2 cups roughly chopped dandelion green leaves
- 2 cups chopped green leaf lettuce leaves
- 2 cups chopped watercress leaves
- 1 medium yellow onion, diced
- 8 cloves garlic, sliced thin
- 5 cups homemade chicken broth
- 2 tsp lemon juice
- 1 tbsp sea salt

METHOD

1 In a medium stockpot, combine baby spinach, Swiss chard, dandelion greens, green leaf lettuce, watercress, yellow onion, garlic, and chicken broth. Set over high heat, and bring to a boil.

2 Reduce heat to medium-low, and simmer, uncovered, for 10 minutes or until leaves are softened.

3 Add lemon juice and sea salt, and stir into soup until combined.

4 If not serving immediately, place the pot in the sink and surround with cold water and ice cubes to cool soup quickly.

5 Refrigerate tightly covered for up to 1 week, or freeze for up to 6 months.

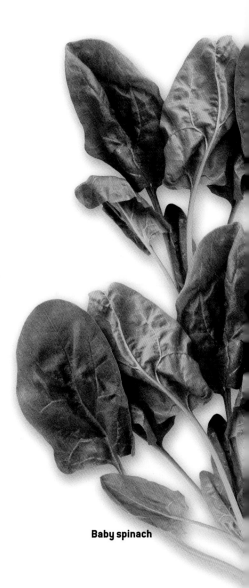
Baby spinach

DAIRY FREE

NUT FREE

PALEO DIET

Sweet-and-Sour Chicken Vegetable Soup

Earthy Asian vegetables star in this fragrant, brothy soup that's ideal for leftover stock chicken. Now chicken soup's not only good for the soul; it's great for the gut, too.

Prep Time
15 minutes

Cook Time
20 minutes

Makes
8 cups

Serving Size
2 cups

INGREDIENTS

- 4 cups homemade chicken stock
- 2 cups cooked chicken (left over from making stock)
- 2 cloves garlic, sliced
- 2 tsp fresh grated ginger
- 1 medium scallion, green and white parts, chopped
- 1 medium yellow onion, peeled, chopped
- 1 medium red bell pepper, ribs and seeds removed, and chopped
- 1 cup thinly sliced shitake mushroom caps
- $1/2$ cup chopped broccoli florets
- $1/2$ cup peeled and thinly sliced carrots
- 1 tsp sea salt
- 2 tbsp raw honey
- $1/4$ cup lemon or fermented vegetable juice

METHOD

1 In a medium stockpot, combine chicken stock, chicken, garlic, ginger, scallion, yellow onion, red bell pepper, shitake mushrooms, broccoli, carrots, and sea salt. Set over medium-high heat, and bring to a boil.

2 Cover, reduce heat to medium-low, and simmer for 20 minutes or until vegetables are just softened.

3 Uncover, and stir in honey and lemon juice.

> If fresh shitakes aren't available, substitute cremini or brown button mushrooms, stem on and sliced thin.

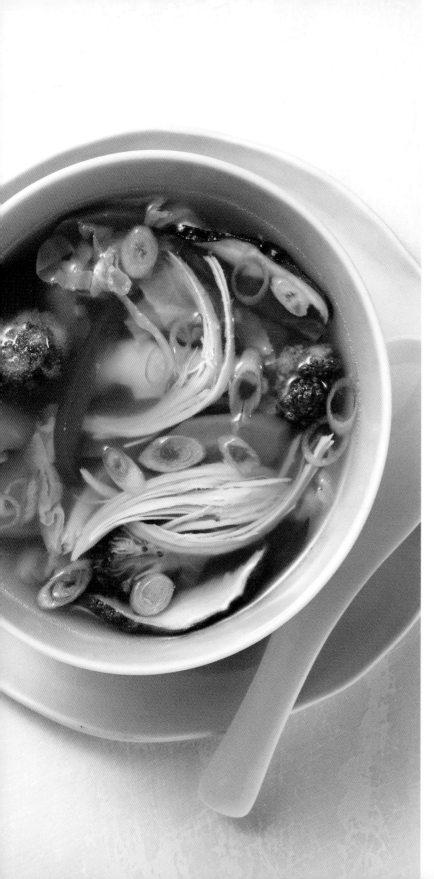

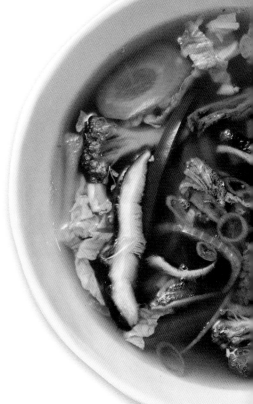

Variation

Sweet-and-Sour Beef Vegetable Soup

Substitute 4 cups beef stock and 4 cups cooked beef shank (from making stock) for the chicken stock and cooked chicken.

STAGE 1

DAIRY FREE

NUT FREE

PALEO DIET

Summer Garden Soup

This fresh, hearty soup captures the variety of the summer growing season in a bowl. It's a true melting pot of garden goodness.

Prep Time	Cook Time	Makes	Serving Size
10 minutes	30 minutes	10 cups	2 cups

INGREDIENTS

- 4 cups homemade chicken stock
- 4 cloves garlic, chopped
- 1 medium yellow onion, chopped
- 1 medium carrot, peeled and cut into $1/2$-in (1.25cm) rounds
- 1 small yellow squash, cut into $1/2$-in (1.25cm) rounds
- 1 small zucchini, cut into $1/2$-in (1.25cm) rounds
- 1 medium red bell pepper, ribs and seeds removed, and chopped
- 2 medium red ripe tomatoes, chopped
- $1/2$ cup fresh green beans, cut into 1-in (2.5cm) pieces
- 2 tsp fresh lemon juice
- 2 tsp sea salt

METHOD

1 In a medium stockpot, combine chicken stock, garlic, yellow onion, carrot, yellow squash, zucchini, red bell pepper, tomatoes, green beans, lemon juice, and sea salt. Set over high heat, and bring to a boil.

2 Reduce heat to medium-low, and simmer, uncovered, for 25 minutes or until vegetables are tender.

3 If not serving immediately, place the pot in the sink and surround with cold water and ice cubes to cool soup quickly.

4 Refrigerate tightly covered for up to 1 week.

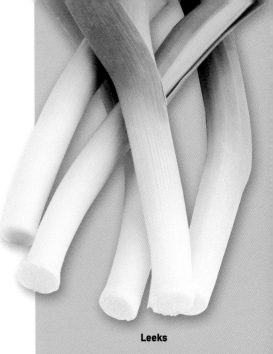
Leeks

Variation

Winter Garden Soup

STAGE 1

Use 4 cloves chopped garlic, 1 cup chopped white part of leeks, 1 medium peeled and chopped carrot, 2 cups cremini mushrooms, 1 cup peeled and diced turnip, 2 cups peeled and diced butternut squash, 2 teaspoons lemon juice, 2 teaspoons sea salt, and 5 cups homemade chicken stock. Proceed as directed.

DAIRY FREE

NUT FREE

PALEO DIET

Three-Onion Soup

This onion, scallion, and garlic soup is beefy and salty. In later stages, you can top a bowl with a slice of toasted grain-free bread and grated Parmesan cheese for a gut-healthy twist on the traditional French classic.

Prep Time
10 minutes

Cook Time
30 minutes

Makes
8 cups

Serving Size
2 cups

INGREDIENTS

- 4 medium scallions, white and green parts, cut thin on the diagonal
- 4 cloves garlic, sliced thin
- 2 medium yellow onions, halved and sliced thin
- 6 cups homemade beef stock
- 1 bay leaf
- 1 tbsp sea salt

METHOD

1 In a medium stockpot, combine scallions, garlic, yellow onions, beef stock, bay leaf, and sea salt. Set over high heat, and bring to a boil.

2 Reduce heat to medium-low, and simmer, uncovered, for 25 minutes. Remove bay leaf.

3 If not serving immediately, place the pot in the sink and surround with cold water and ice cubes to cool soup quickly.

4 Refrigerate tightly covered for up to 1 week.

If the onions, garlic, and scallions aren't enough onion flavor for you, you can add 3 medium shallots, halved and sliced thin.

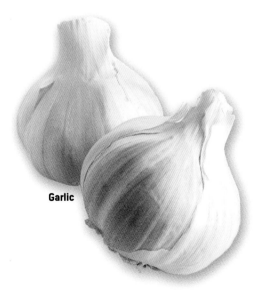
Garlic

NUT FREE

Pumpkin Bisque

Simple yet decadent, this smooth purée highlights pumpkin, an often-overlooked nutritional overachiever in the winter squash family. A dollop of creamy, probiotic-rich homemade yogurt makes this soup perfect for chilly autumn weather.

Prep Time	Cook Time	Makes	Serving Size
10 minutes	20 minutes	4 cups	1 cup

INGREDIENTS

- 2 medium sugar pumpkins, split, seeded, peeled, and cubed
- 1 medium yellow onion, chopped
- 1 clove garlic, chopped
- 2 fresh shiitake mushroom caps, chopped
- ¹/₂ tsp sea salt
- 1 tsp lemon juice
- 5 cups homemade chicken stock
- ¹/₄ cup homemade yogurt
- 2 tbsp ghee

METHOD

1 In a large stockpot, combine sugar pumpkins, yellow onion, garlic, shiitake mushrooms, sea salt, lemon juice, and chicken stock. Set over medium-high heat, and bring to a boil.

2 Cover, reduce heat to medium-low, and simmer for about 20 minutes or until squash is softened.

3 Working in small batches, purée soup in a blender.

4 Serve with a dollop of homemade yogurt and a drizzle of ghee.

If you can't find sugar pumpkins, substitute 1 (15-ounce; 420g) can organic pumpkin purée with no added ingredients. To make this soup low FODMAP, omit the onion and garlic, use oyster or chanterelle mushrooms if you can't find fresh shiitake, and limit the serving size to ¹/₃ cup. This might alter the flavor of the finished dish, so use your best judgment and what feels right for your gut.

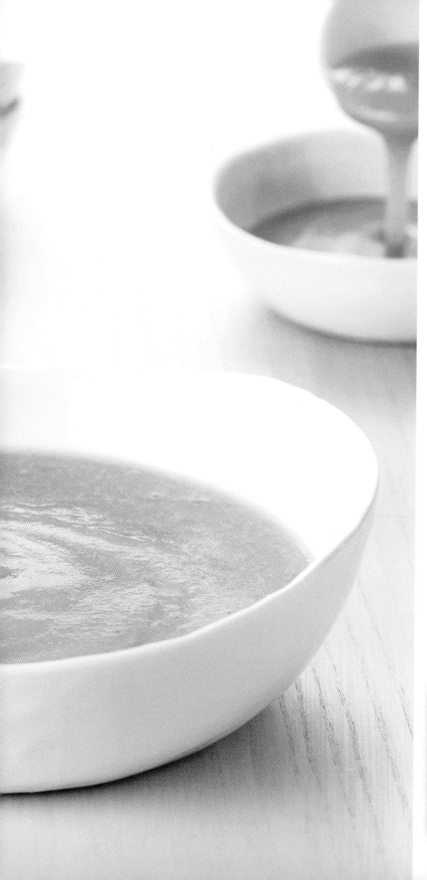

Variation

Roasted Pumpkin Bisque

Substitute 3 cups roasted pumpkin purée for sugar pumpkins, and add 1 teaspoon pumpkin pie spice. Cook and purée as directed, and garnish each serving with 1 tablespoon homemade yogurt and 1 teaspoon ghee.

STAGE 4

Component

Roasted Pumpkin

STAGE 4

METHOD

1 Preheat the oven to 375°F (190°C). Lightly grease a baking sheet with ghee.

2 Split pumpkin in half, place flesh side down on the prepared baking sheet, and roast for 30 minutes or until tender when poked with a knife.

3 Allow pumpkin to cool to the touch, and scoop out and discard seeds with a spoon.

4 Scoop out and reserve roasted pumpkin flesh. Discard skin.

Roasted pumpkin

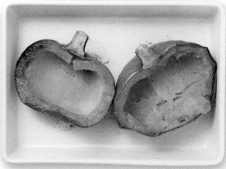

**NUT
FREE**

Creamy Tomato Soup

With a fresh, fruity taste and fragrance, this bright red soup is
very versatile. Serve it warm soup during cold months, or use your
garden fresh tomatoes and serve it chilled when the weather is hot.

Prep Time	Cook Time	Makes	Serving Size
10 minutes	20 minutes	8 cups	2 cups

INGREDIENTS

- 6 medium fresh ripe red
  tomatoes, chopped
- 1 medium yellow onion,
  chopped
- 2 cloves garlic, chopped
- 5 cups homemade chicken
  stock
- 2 tsp sea salt
- 1 cup homemade yogurt
  (as tolerated)

METHOD

1 In a medium stockpot, combine
tomatoes, yellow onion, garlic,
chicken stock, and sea salt. Set over high
heat, and bring to a boil.

2 Reduce heat to medium-low, cover,
and simmer for 15 minutes.

3 Remove from heat, uncover, and
working in small batches, purée
soup in a blender until smooth. Or use
an immersion blender.

4 If you can tolerate dairy, top each
bowl with $1/4$ cup homemade yogurt
before serving.

> Puréeing hot soup can cause scalding burns.
> Fill the blender less than half full, add the lid
> but remove the center knob, cover the lid and
> hole with a folded kitchen towel, and press
> down to secure before blending.

Tomatoes

DAIRY FREE

NUT FREE

PALEO DIET

Greek Lemon Vegetable Soup

Lemon shines alongside a variety of hearty vegetables in this traditional Greek soup. Grated cauliflower floret "rice" provides the appeal of rice without the grain.

Prep Time
10 minutes

Cook Time
20 minutes

Makes
8 cups

Serving Size
2 cups

INGREDIENTS

1 cup cooked and shredded chicken (from making stock)

3 cloves garlic, chopped

1 medium yellow onion, diced

1 medium carrot, peeled and sliced thin

$1/2$ tsp sea salt

4 cups homemade chicken stock

$1/4$ cup fresh lemon juice

2 tbsp animal fat (or ghee if dairy is tolerated)

1 cup grated cauliflower florets

2 medium red ripe tomatoes, chopped

2 cups chopped baby spinach

2 sprigs Italian flat-leaf parsley

METHOD

1 In a medium stockpot, combine chicken, garlic, yellow onion, carrot, sea salt, and chicken stock. Set over medium-high heat, and bring to a boil.

2 Reduce heat to medium-low, cover, and cook for 20 minutes or until vegetables are softened. Remove from heat.

3 Add lemon juice and animal fat.

4 Add cauliflower, tomatoes, baby spinach, and Italian flat-leaf parsley, and stir to combine for 3 minutes until vegetables are softened. Remove parsley sprigs before serving.

To make this soup low FODMAP, omit the onion and garlic.

Variation

Lemon Vegetable "Rice" Soup

STAGE 3

You can create a subtle, creamy variation of this soup:

1 Whisk 2 large pastured whole eggs in a medium bowl until frothy. Slowly whisk 1 cup finished warm soup into egg mixture. When combined, slowly whisk in another cup of soup.

2 Transfer the egg mixture back into the larger soup pot, stirring regularly. Replace the parsley sprigs with $1/4$ cup chopped Italian flat-leaf parsley, folded into the soup after the egg mixture is added.

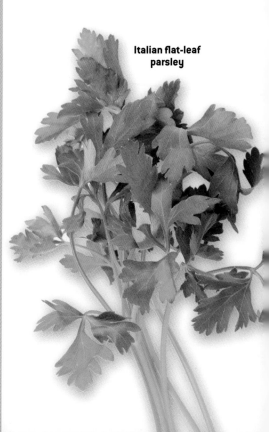
Italian flat-leaf parsley

DAIRY
FREE

NUT
FREE

PALEO
DIET

Beet and Beef Short Rib Borscht

This soup is full of vibrantly colored beets; softened, flavorful vegetables; and tender, juicy short ribs. Even people who don't like beets will like this.

Prep Time
20 minutes

Cook Time
2 hours

Makes
12 cups

Serving Size
2 cups

INGREDIENTS

2 bay leaves

1 bunch fresh thyme

4 whole black peppercorns

4 bone-in short ribs (about 4 lb; 2kg)

1 tsp sea salt

2 cloves garlic, sliced thin

1¼ cups tomato purée

4 cups homemade beef stock

1 medium yellow onion, chopped into ½-in (1.25cm) pieces

3 medium carrots, peeled and chopped into ½-in (1.25cm) pieces

3 medium red ripe tomatoes, cored and chopped into ½-in (1.25cm) pieces

4 medium beets, peeled and chopped into ½-in (1.25cm) pieces

¼ cup fermented vegetable juice

¼ cup homemade yogurt (optional)

METHOD

1. Preheat the oven to 375°F (190°C). Bundle bay leaves, thyme, and black peppercorns in a piece of cheesecloth, and tie tightly closed.

2. Season short ribs with sea salt, and place in a medium stockpot. Add garlic, tomato purée, beef stock, and cheesecloth bundle. Cover, and cook on the middle oven rack for 1 hour.

3. Remove from the oven, and add yellow onion, carrots, tomatoes, and beets. Cover, return to the oven, and cook for 1 hour or until vegetables and short ribs are tender.

4. Remove from the oven, and remove and discard cheesecloth bundle.

5. Pull shredded beef from bones, and return to the pot. Fold in fermented vegetable juice.

6. Garnish individual portions with homemade yogurt (if using), and serve.

> To make this dish low FODMAP, omit the onion and garlic.

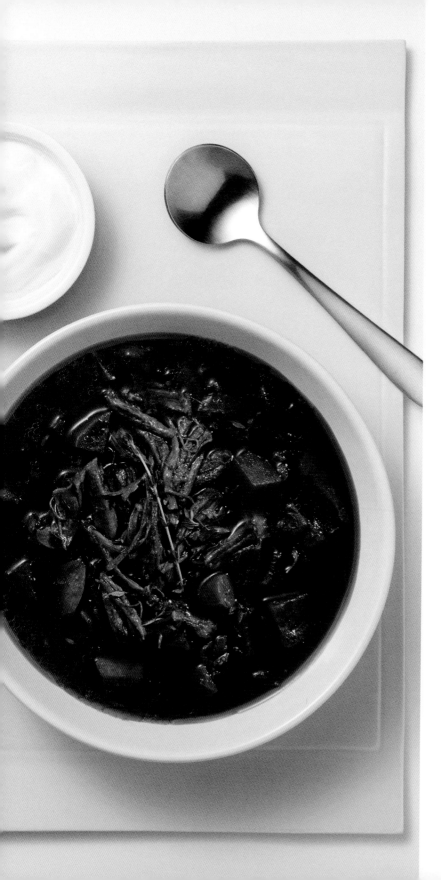

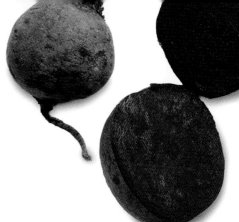

Beets

Variation

Slow Cooker Beet and Beef Short Rib Borscht

Increase the homemade beef stock to 6 cups and combine stock, short ribs, sea salt, garlic, tomato purée, yellow onion, carrots, tomatoes, beets, and cheesecloth bundle in a 4-quart (4-liter) slow cooker. Cover and cook on low for 8 hours. Transfer cooked short ribs to a plate, and remove beef from bones. Return beef to the cooker, and fold in fermented vegetable juice. Remove and discard cheesecloth bundle, garnish individual portions with homemade yogurt (if using), and serve.

STAGE 1

NUT FREE   LOW FODMAP   PALEO DIET

Stewed Beef Porridge

The meat, fat, and connective tissue left over from making stock or bone broth is nourishing and easy on the gut. This recipe yields a quick, tasty breakfast that fills and fuels you while saving money by using leftover meat.

Prep Time
5 minutes

Cook Time
10 to 12 minutes

Makes
1 cup

Serving Size
1 cup

INGREDIENTS

1 cup meat, fat, and connective tissue reserved from making broth or stock

$^{1}/_{2}$ cup homemade beef stock or broth

1 or 2 tsp animal fat or coconut oil (or ghee if dairy is tolerated)

Sea salt

METHOD

1 In a blender, pulse meat, fat, connective tissue, and beef stock 2 or 3 times or until your desired consistency.

2 Transfer purée to small saucepan, set over medium heat, and cook for 5 to 7 minutes.

3 Add animal fat, and cook for 5 minutes or until fat is melted and combined.

4 Season with sea salt, and serve immediately.

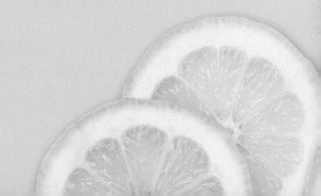

DAIRY FREE **NUT FREE** **LOW FODMAP** **PALEO DIET**

Lemon Peppercorn Poached Chicken Breast

Infusing rich chicken stock with even more aromatics produces a tangy, slightly peppery chicken dish. In later stages, add fresh ginger, sliced orange, star anise, cilantro, or even saffron to the poaching liquid.

Prep Time	Cook Time	Makes	Serving Size
10 minutes	20 minutes	4 chicken breasts	1 breast

INGREDIENTS

4 sprigs thyme

1 bay leaf

1 tsp whole black peppercorns

4 cups homemade chicken stock

1/4 cup fresh lemon juice

1 medium lemon, sliced

1 tsp sea salt

4 (6-oz; 170g) boneless, skinless chicken breasts

METHOD

1 Bundle thyme, bay leaf, and black peppercorns in a piece of cheesecloth, and tightly tie closed.

2 In a large, deep skillet, combine chicken stock, lemon juice, lemon slices, cheesecloth bundle, and sea salt. Set over high heat, and bring to a boil.

3 Add chicken breasts, and cook for 3 minutes. Remove from heat, cover, and set aside for 15 minutes.

4 Remove and discard sliced lemon and cheesecloth bundle.

5 If using immediately, remove chicken from the skillet and serve. If not using immediately, refrigerate cooled chicken tightly covered for up to 1 week.

To reheat leftover poached chicken breasts, place in a skillet over medium-high heat with 1/4 cup homemade chicken stock per breast. Bring to a boil, reduce heat to medium-low, cover, and simmer for 5 minutes or until chicken is warmed through.

Lemon slices

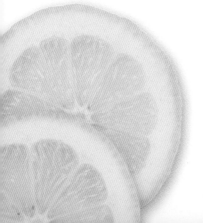

DAIRY FREE

NUT FREE

PALEO DIET

Pan Steak with Mushrooms

Earthy mushrooms and tender sliced beef pair well with a side dish of creamy Cauliflower Mash. This is great for the meat-and-potato lover, or anyone looking for a warm and hearty stage 1 meal.

Prep Time	Cook Time	Makes	Serving Size
15 minutes	20 minutes	4 steaks + 2 cups sauce	1 steak + $^1/_2$ cup sauce

INGREDIENTS

8 whole black peppercorns

1 sprig thyme

1 (1-lb; 450g) skirt or New York strip steak

$^1/_2$ tsp sea salt

2 cloves garlic, sliced

$^1/_2$ cup diced small yellow onion

1 cup fresh shiitake mushrooms, stems removed and cut in half

1 cup brown button or cremini mushrooms

2 cups homemade beef stock

METHOD

1 Bundle black peppercorns and thyme in a piece of cheesecloth, and tightly tie closed.

2 Season skirt steak on both sides with sea salt, and place in a large skillet. Add garlic, yellow onion, shiitake mushrooms, button mushrooms, beef stock, and cheesecloth bundle. Set heat to medium-high, and bring to a boil.

3 Cover, reduce heat to medium-low, and simmer for 20 minutes or until internal temperature of steak reaches 140°F (60°C) for medium.

4 Remove steak from the skillet, and allow to rest for 10 minutes. Cut into 4 equal-size pieces.

5 Remove and discard cheesecloth bundle, and serve steak with sauce over top.

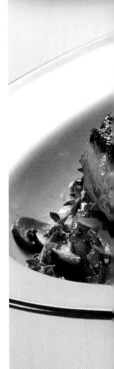

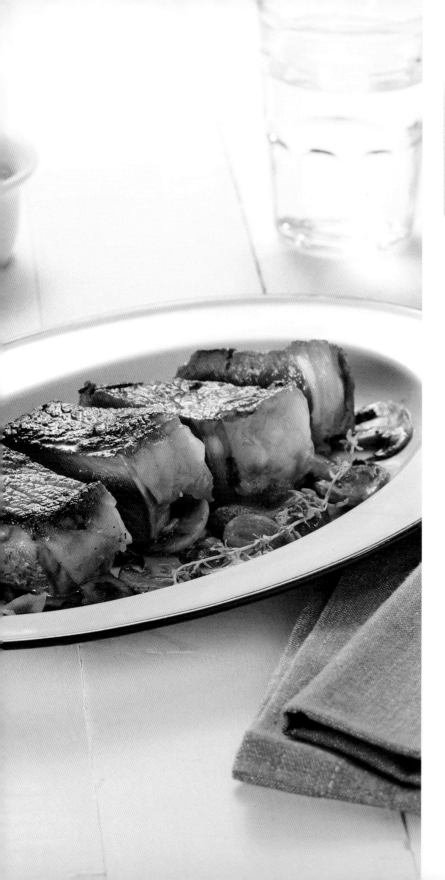

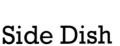

Side Dish

Cauliflower Mash

You'll never miss the potatoes when you pair your steak with this healthy comfort dish, which you can make while the steak is cooking.

INGREDIENTS
1 medium head cauliflower
½ tsp sea salt
¼ cup ghee

METHOD
1 Core cauliflower and cut into small florets. Place in a steamer basket in a large saucepan. Add ½ inch (1.25cm) water, set over medium-high heat, and bring to a boil. Cover, reduce heat to medium-low, and simmer for 10 minutes or until florets are soft and fork-tender.

2 Drain in a colander, pressing out any excess water. Add cauliflower to a food processor fitted with a metal chopping blade, add sea salt and ghee, and process until smooth.

STAGE 1

STAGE 2

STAGE 3

STAGE 4

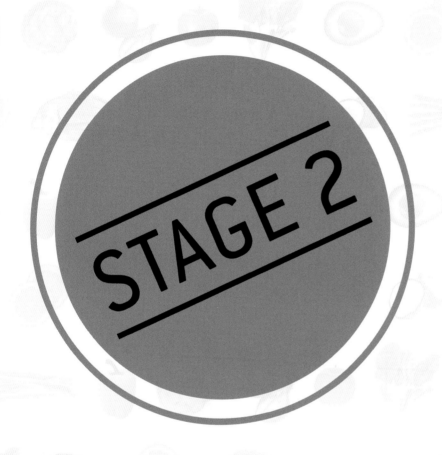

STAGE 2

STAGE 5

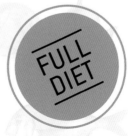

STAGE 6

FULL
DIET

DAIRY FREE

NUT FREE

PALEO DIET

Egg Drop Soup

Light, silky egg flowers complement perfectly salty broth, tender and meaty shiitake mushrooms, sweet green onions, and just-spicy-enough ginger in this traditional Chinese super soup.

Prep Time	Cook Time	Makes	Serving Size
10 minutes	15 minutes	8 cups	2 cups

INGREDIENTS

- 2 tbsp animal fat (or ghee if dairy is tolerated)
- 6 cups homemade chicken stock
- 2 cups sliced fresh shiitake mushrooms, stems removed
- 1 cup thinly sliced scallions, white and green parts
- 2 cloves garlic, minced
- 1 tsp grated fresh ginger
- 1 tbsp sea salt
- 6 egg whites, or 3 whole eggs if yolks are tolerated well

METHOD

1 In a medium stockpot, combine animal fat, chicken stock, shiitake mushrooms, scallions, garlic, ginger, and sea salt. Set over medium-high heat, and bring to a boil.

2 Reduce heat to medium-low, and simmer, uncovered, for 15 minutes.

3 Turn heat off, and gently drizzle in egg yolks while stirring broth slowly.

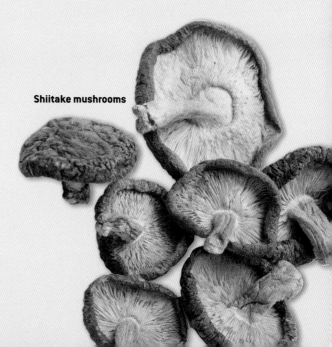

Shiitake mushrooms

If you're out of chicken or want a different flavor, you can substitute beef or fish stock. If fresh shiitakes aren't available, substitute an equal amount of brown button or cremini mushrooms.

DAIRY FREE   **NUT FREE**   **PALEO DIET**

Vegetable Beef Stewp

A cross between a soup and a stew, this bold one-pot dish features soft, chunky vegetables and mouthwatering, easy-to-digest beef rich in protein and minerals like zinc and iron, all swimming in a gravylike broth.

Prep Time	Cook Time	Makes	Serving Size
15 minutes	45 minutes	8 cups	2 cups

INGREDIENTS

1 lb (450g) beef stew meat

2 medium yellow onions, chopped

2 medium carrots, peeled and chopped

1 cup chopped tomatoes

1 clove garlic, chopped fine

1 bay leaf

3 sprigs thyme leaves, chopped fine

1 tbsp lemon juice

1 tsp sea salt

4 cups homemade beef stock

$^1/_4$ cup fresh Italian flat-leaf parsley

METHOD

1 In a large stockpot, combine beef, yellow onions, carrots, tomatoes, garlic, bay leaf, thyme, lemon juice, and sea salt. Pour in beef stock, set over medium-high heat, and bring to a boil.

2 Cover, reduce heat to medium-low, and simmer for 45 minutes or until beef and vegetables are tender.

3 Fold in Italian flat-leaf parsley, and remove bay leaf. If sauce isn't thick enough, uncover and continue to cook until sauce thickens to your liking.

To make this dish low FODMAP, omit the onions and garlic and limit the serving size to $^1/_3$ cup.

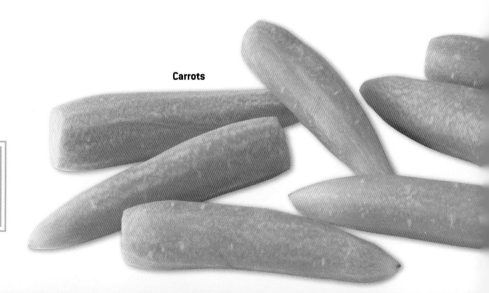

Carrots

DAIRY FREE

NUT FREE

PALEO DIET

Braised Beef Burgers

These warm and juicy braised beef burgers, with onions, mushrooms, and tomatoes, feature a fragrant, hearty gravy. It's comforting on a cold evening. You can serve them in a bowl topped with sauce, or put them on grain-free bread for a juicy version of the typical burger. Either way, they're hearty and satisfying.

Prep Time
15 minutes

Cook Time
10 minutes

Makes
4 burgers + 2 cups sauce

Serving Size
1 burger + ¹/₂ cup sauce

INGREDIENTS

1 lb (450g) ground beef

1 tsp sea salt

1 tbsp lard or coconut oil (or ghee if dairy is tolerated)

2 cloves garlic, chopped

2 cups sliced brown button mushrooms

¹/₂ cup diced yellow onion

1 cup diced tomatoes

1 cup homemade beef stock

1 tbsp chopped fresh thyme leaves

1 tbsp chopped fresh Italian flat-leaf parsley

METHOD

1 Form ground beef into 4 (1-inch-; 2.5cm-thick) patties, and season evenly with sea salt.

2 Place patties in a large skillet. Add lard or coconut oil, garlic, brown button mushrooms, yellow onion, tomatoes, beef stock, thyme, and Italian flat-leaf parsley. Set heat to high, and bring to a boil.

3 Cover, reduce heat to medium-low, and cook for 10 minutes or until beef is cooked through and no pink remains in center of patties.

4 Remove from heat, and serve patties in a bowl topped with sauce.

> To make this dish low FODMAP, omit the onion and garlic and use oyster, chanterelle, or shiitake mushrooms instead.

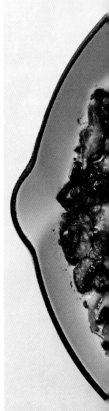

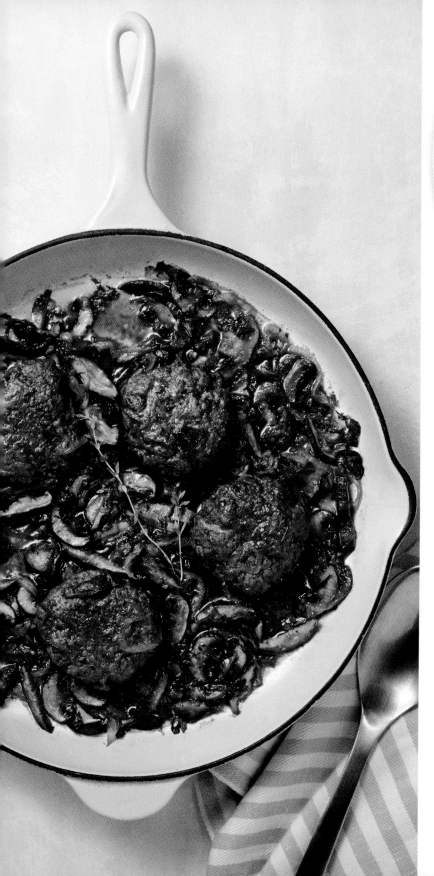

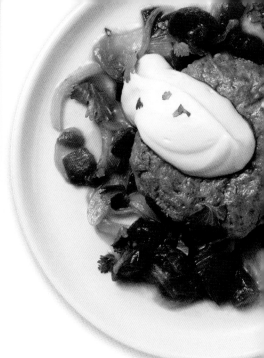

Variation

Mexicali Turkey Burgers

Substitute ground turkey for the beef and chicken stock for the beef stock. Omit the brown button mushrooms, substitute red onion for the yellow onion and 2 tablespoons fresh chopped cilantro leaves for the thyme, add 1 extra cup chopped tomatoes and 1 tablespoon fresh lemon juice, and cook as directed for 15 minutes or until no pink remains in center of patties and internal temperature is 165°F (75°C). Top with 1 tablespoon homemade yogurt. In stage 3, you can add ¼ fresh avocado.

STAGE 2

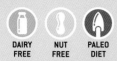

DAIRY FREE **NUT FREE** **PALEO DIET**

Asian Braised Turkey Meatballs

These meatballs might not be exactly like your grandma's, but they're warm, juicy, and surrounded by satisfying flavors.

Prep Time
15 minutes

Cook Time
30 minutes

Makes
32 meatballs

Serving Size
8 meatballs

INGREDIENTS

2 lb (1kg) ground turkey thighs

4 large egg yolks

1 tbsp sea salt

2 tbsp animal fat (or ghee if dairy is tolerated)

4 cups homemade chicken stock

3 cups tomato purée

3 tbsp fresh lemon juice

1 tbsp grated fresh ginger

4 cloves garlic, minced

2 cups chopped scallions, white and green parts

1 medium red onion, halved and sliced

1 medium red bell pepper, halved, ribs and seeds removed, and sliced

1 medium yellow bell pepper, halved, ribs and seeds removed, and sliced

1 medium carrot, peeled and cut into $^1/_2$-in (1.25cm) rounds

$^1/_2$ cup chopped fresh cilantro leaves

METHOD

1 In a medium bowl, combine ground turkey, egg yolks, and $1^1/_2$ teaspoons sea salt. Form mixture into 32 equal-size balls.

2 In a medium Dutch oven or stockpot, combine animal fat, chicken stock, tomato purée, lemon juice, ginger, garlic, scallions, red onion, red bell pepper, yellow bell pepper, carrot, cilantro, and remaining $1^1/_2$ teaspoon sea salt. Set over medium-high heat, and bring to a boil.

3 Reduce heat to medium-low, and gently add meatballs to the pot one by one. Cover, and cook for 30 minutes or until meatballs are cooked through and no pink remains.

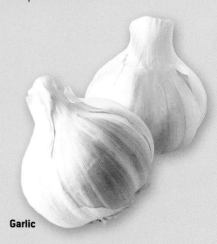

Garlic

DAIRY
FREE

NUT
FREE

PALEO
DIET

Ground Chicken Stuffed Cabbage Rolls

These little rolls are filled with warm and juicy chicken, wrapped in a softened cabbage shell, and covered with a yummy tomato broth.

Prep Time
30 minutes

Cook Time
30 minutes

Makes
8 rolls

Serving Size
2 rolls

INGREDIENTS

2 qt (2 liters) water

8 large green cabbage leaves

2 lb (1kg) ground chicken

1 large yellow onion

4 cloves garlic, minced

4 cups homemade chicken stock

1 1/2 cups grated cauliflower

2 tbsp animal fat (or ghee if dairy is tolerated)

4 cups tomato purée

2 bay leaves

1 tbsp sea salt

METHOD

1 In a medium stockpot over high heat, bring water to a boil. Reduce heat to medium-low, add green cabbage, and press leaves into water using a spoon. Cover, and cook for 10 minutes or until soft. Remove cabbage from the pot, drain, and set aside to cool.

2 In the pot, combine chicken, yellow onion, garlic, and 2 cups chicken stock. Set over medium-high heat, and bring to a boil. Reduce heat to medium-low, cover, and simmer for 15 minutes or until chicken is cooked. Fold in grated cauliflower until combined.

3 Place 1 softened cabbage leaf, curve side up with stem facing you, on a plate. Add 3/4 cup ground chicken mixture on stem end. Fold in sides about 1 inch (2.5cm), and roll stem end away until completely rolled. Repeat with remaining leaves and filling.

4 In a medium Dutch oven or stockpot, combine animal fat, remaining 2 cups chicken stock, tomato purée, bay leaves, and sea salt. Add cabbage rolls, seam side down.

5 Set over medium-high heat, and bring to a boil. Reduce heat to medium-low, cover, and simmer for 30 minutes. Remove bay leaves, and serve.

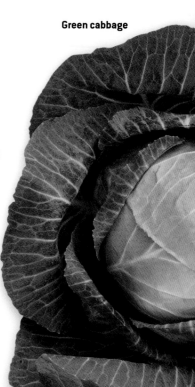

Green cabbage

DAIRY FREE

NUT FREE

PALEO DIET

Chicken Vegetable Ratatouille

Hearty and comforting, this colorful, vegetable-based stew is tasty cold or hot, depending on your preference. The Mediterranean influence captures the nourishing bounty of the summer season in one pot.

Prep Time	**Cook Time**	**Makes**	**Serving Size**
15 minutes	1 hour	4 cups + 4 legs	1 cup + 1 leg

INGREDIENTS

4 skin-on, bone-in chicken leg quarters (about 2 lb; 1kg)

1 tsp sea salt

4 cups homemade chicken stock

$^3/_4$ cup diced yellow onion

4 cloves garlic, sliced

$^3/_4$ cup diced green bell pepper

2 cups diced Italian eggplant, skin on

$1^1/_2$ cups diced zucchini, skin on

$1^1/_2$ cups diced yellow summer squash, skin on

2 cups diced tomatoes

$^1/_4$ cup chopped fresh Italian flat-leaf parsley

$^1/_4$ cup chopped fresh basil leaves

$^1/_4$ cup animal fat (or ghee if dairy is tolerated)

METHOD

1. Place chicken leg quarters in a large, deep skillet, and season with sea salt. Add chicken stock to cover $^2/_3$ of chicken. Set heat to medium-high.

2. When stock begins to simmer, cover, reduce heat to medium-low, and simmer for 45 minutes or until chicken legs are cooked through to an internal temperature of 165°F (75°C).

3. Add yellow onion, garlic, green bell pepper, Italian eggplant, zucchini, yellow summer squash, and tomatoes. Cover and cook for 15 more minutes.

4. Remove from heat. Add Italian flat-leaf parsley, basil, and animal fat, and stir.

Prevent food-borne illness by cooking the chicken to an internal temperature of at least 165°F (75°C) as measured on a calibrated food thermometer. To make this dish low FODMAP, omit the onion and garlic.

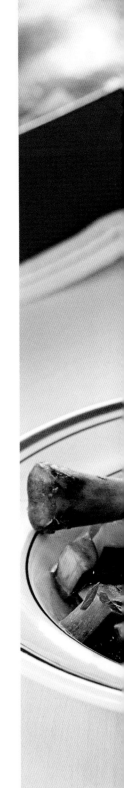

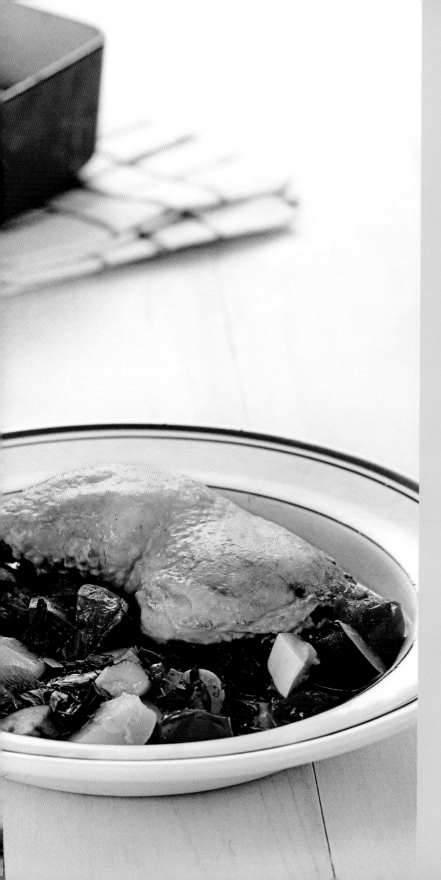

Variation

Winter Ratatouille

STAGE 2

In place of the ingredients in step 3, substitute the following:

4 cloves garlic, chopped

1 cup chopped leeks, white part only

1 medium carrot, peeled and sliced into rounds

2 cups halved cremini mushrooms

2 cups peeled, seeded, and diced butternut squash

2 cups chopped red ripe tomatoes

2 tsp lemon juice

Increase the cook time to 20 minutes, and continue with step 4.

DAIRY FREE **NUT FREE** **PALEO DIET**

Chicken Enchilada Casserole

This tasty and refreshing south-of-the-border one-pot is easy to assemble. Build flavor as you move through the diet by adding avocado in stage 3 and ground cumin in stage 5.

Prep Time
15 minutes

Cook Time
50 minutes

Makes
8 thighs

Serving Size
2 thighs

INGREDIENTS

4 cups homemade chicken stock

2 cups tomato purée

1 cup chopped tomatoes

1 cup chopped red bell pepper

2 cloves garlic, chopped

1 cup chopped red onion

1 cup chopped scallions, green and white parts

$^1/_2$ cup lime juice

$^1/_2$ cup chopped fresh cilantro leaves

2 tsp sea salt

8 bone-in, skin-on chicken thighs (about 3 lb; 1.5kg)

1 cup homemade yogurt (optional)

METHOD

1 In a medium Dutch oven, combine chicken stock, tomato purée, tomatoes, red bell pepper, garlic, red onion, scallions, lime juice, cilantro, and sea salt.

2 Add chicken thighs on top of vegetables so chicken skin is just peeking out of top of broth. Set over medium-high heat, and bring to a boil.

3 Reduce heat to medium-low, cover, and cook for 30 minutes.

4 Preheat the oven to 350°F (180°C). Uncover Dutch oven, transfer to the oven, and cook for 10 minutes.

5 Set oven to broil, and broil for 5 minutes or until chicken skin is browned.

6 Serve with a dollop of homemade yogurt (if using) on each bowl.

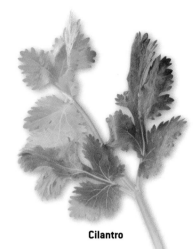

Cilantro

Variations

Avocado Enchiladas

STAGE 3

In stage 3, you can add guacamole to the toppings, too.

Spicy Chicken Enchilada Casserole

STAGE 5

In stage 5, you can pump up the flavor by adding ground cumin in step 1.

DAIRY FREE **NUT FREE** **PALEO DIET**

Lemon Rosemary Salmon

This simple recipe yields a moist, clean, and light finished fillet with the aroma of fresh lemon and fragrant rosemary. Make extra, allow to cool, and use flaked in omelets and on salads.

Prep Time
10 minutes

Cook Time
10 minutes

Makes
4 fillets

Serving Size
1 fillet

INGREDIENTS

- 1 tsp sea salt
- 2 lb (1kg) wild salmon, with skin, cut into 4 (8-oz; 225g) fillets
- 2 sprigs thyme
- 4 sprigs rosemary
- 1/4 cup fresh lemon juice
- 1 medium lemon, sliced
- 4 cloves garlic, chopped
- 1/2 medium yellow onion, sliced thin
- 6 cups homemade fish or chicken stock

To make this dish low FODMAP, omit the onion and garlic.

METHOD

1 Sprinkle sea salt evenly over salmon.

2 In a skillet large enough to hold salmon in a single layer without touching, combine thyme, rosemary, lemon juice, lemon slices, garlic, yellow onion, and fish stock. Set over medium-high heat, and bring to a boil.

3 Reduce heat to medium-low, add salmon, cover, and cook for 5 minutes or until salmon is cooked through.

4 Divide salmon evenly among 4 bowls. Strain stock through a fine-mesh strainer into a large pan, and pour 1 cup stock over each piece.

5 If not serving immediately, allow salmon to cool completely, remove from stock, and refrigerate tightly covered for up to 1 week. Strain stock, and refrigerate for up to 1 week or freeze for up to 6 months.

Variation

Lemon and Rosemary Butter-Poached Salmon

1 Replace fish stock with 4 cups ghee.

STAGE 4

2 In a large skillet over medium-low heat, cook ghee, thyme, rosemary, lemon juice, lemon slices, garlic, and yellow onion for about 8 minutes or until small bubbles begin to appear.

3 Add salmon, and cook for 15 minutes or until top is completely opaque and flakes with a fork. Remove salmon from ghee, and serve.

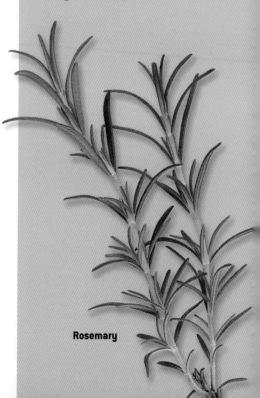

Rosemary

DAIRY FREE **NUT FREE** **PALEO DIET**

Braised Tomato Sage Turkey Legs

Turkey often connotes holiday celebrations, but it can provide great gut support any time of the year. Juicy, moist turkey meat in a rich, deep tomato sauce bursting with earthy, fresh sage provides comfort in every bite.

Prep Time	**Cook Time**	**Makes**	**Serving Size**
20 minutes	1 hour, 15 minutes	2 turkey legs	½ turkey leg

INGREDIENTS

2 turkey legs (about 5 lb; 2.25kg)

½ tsp sea salt

1 medium yellow onion, chopped

4 cloves garlic, chopped

2 medium carrots, peeled and rough chopped

2 medium stalks celery, rough chopped

4 sprigs thyme

6 sprigs sage

2 bay leaves

3 cups homemade chicken stock

2 cups tomato purée

METHOD

1 Preheat the oven to 325°F (170°C). Place turkey legs in a large skillet, and sprinkle with sea salt.

2 Add yellow onion, garlic, carrots, celery, thyme, sage, bay leaves, chicken stock, and tomato purée.

3 Cover, and cook on the middle oven rack for 1 hour, 15 minutes or until turkey legs are cooked through and reach an internal temperature of 165°F (75°C).

4 Remove bay leaves, and allow turkey to rest for 10 minutes before serving.

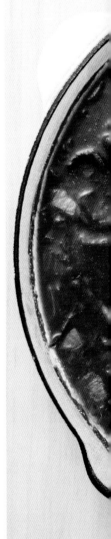

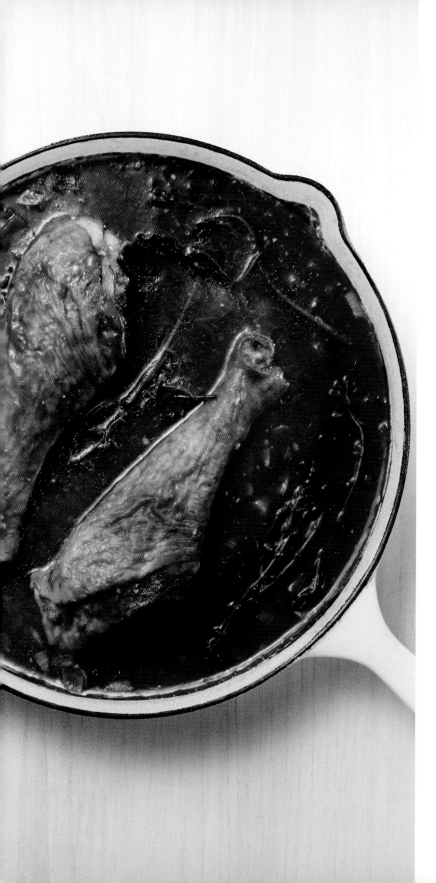

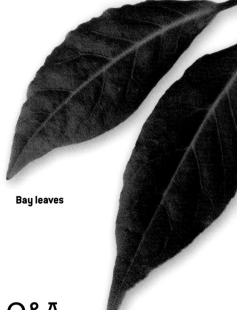

Bay leaves

Q&A

Can I make stock
from the leftover turkey
bones?

Yes you can! Follow the same
steps and ingredients in the
Chicken Stock recipe, but reduce
to 3 quarts (3 liters) water. (Makes
8 cups turkey stock.)

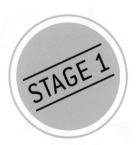

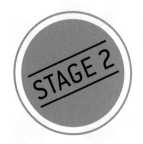

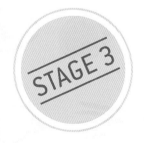

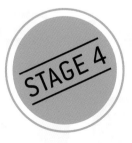

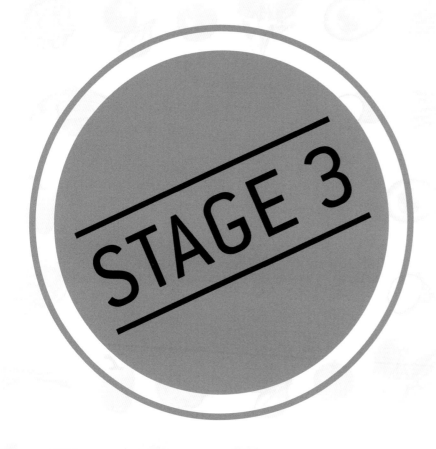

STAGE 3

STAGE 5

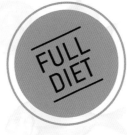

STAGE 6

FULL
DIET

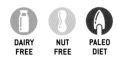

DAIRY FREE **NUT FREE** **PALEO DIET**

Sauerkraut Scramble

Rich, warm eggs and tangy sauerkraut make a lovely pair in this fast and easy scramble. Even the cold leftovers are tasty.

Prep Time
5 minutes

Cook Time
5 minutes

Makes
1 scramble

Serving Size
1 scramble

INGREDIENTS

2 large eggs

2 tbsp water

$1/4$ tsp sea salt

1 tbsp animal fat (or ghee if dairy is tolerated)

$1/4$ cup diced red onion

1 clove garlic, minced

$1/2$ cup Simple Sauerkraut

METHOD

1 In a small bowl, beat eggs, water, and sea salt until blended and foamy.

2 In a medium skillet over medium-high heat, heat animal fat. When hot, add red onion and garlic, and cook, stirring, for about 2 minutes or until soft. Add Simple Sauerkraut, and stir to combine.

3 Pour egg mixture in the center of the skillet. Using a spatula, gently push cooked parts of eggs from the outer edges of the skillet toward the center so uncooked eggs can reach hot skillet surface.

4 Cook for about 2 minutes, gently moving cooked egg portions as needed until top surface of eggs is thickened and no visible liquid egg remains.

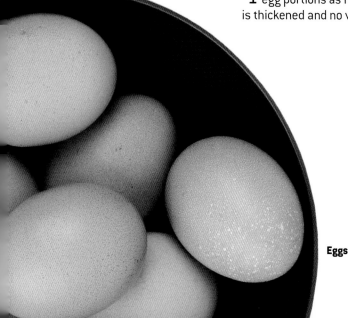

Eggs

NUT FREE

PALEO DIET

Santa Fe Breakfast Tostadas

This tostada is a vibrant tower of delicious veggies, tender chicken, and fresh protein-rich eggs, all topped with smooth, rich avocado mash and tangy homemade yogurt.

Prep Time
15 minutes

Cook Time
7 minutes

Makes
2 tostadas

Serving Size
1 tostada

INGREDIENTS

4 large eggs

4 tbsp ghee or animal fat

1 cup cooked and shredded chicken

1 clove garlic, minced

$^1/_2$ cup sliced red onions

1 cup chopped tomatoes

$^1/_2$ cup chopped scallions, white and green parts

$^1/_2$ cup sliced brown button mushrooms

$^1/_2$ cup peeled and coarsely grated carrots

1 cup zucchini, halved and cut in $^1/_2$-in (1.25cm) half moons

1 cup yellow summer squash, halved and cut in $^1/_2$-in (1.25cm) half moons

$^1/_4$ cup chopped fresh cilantro leaves

$^1/_2$ tsp sea salt

$^1/_2$ cup mashed avocado

$^1/_2$ cup homemade yogurt (optional)

METHOD

1 In a small bowl, whisk eggs until foamy. Heat a medium skillet over medium-high heat.

2 Add 2 tablespoons ghee, chicken, garlic, red onions, tomatoes, scallions, brown button mushrooms, carrots, zucchini, yellow squash, cilantro, and sea salt, and cook, stirring regularly, for 5 minutes or until tender. Transfer to a plate and keep warm.

3 Add remaining 2 tablespoons ghee to the skillet, and pour egg mixture in the center of the skillet. Using a spatula, gently push cooked parts of eggs from the outer edges of the skillet toward the center so uncooked eggs can reach hot skillet surface.

4 Cook for about 2 minutes, gently moving cooked egg portions as needed until top surface of eggs is thickened and no visible liquid egg remains.

5 Divide vegetables between 2 serving plates or bowls. Top each serving with $^1/_2$ of scrambled eggs, $^1/_4$ cup avocado, and $^1/_4$ cup homemade yogurt (if using).

DAIRY FREE

NUT FREE

PALEO DIET

Skillet Asparagus and Eggs

What better way to greet the day than with warm, soft, protein-rich sunny-side-up eggs and buttery, tender-crisp asparagus spears? Even on an elimination diet, breakfast can be the most important meal of the day.

Prep Time
5 minutes

Cook Time
5 minutes

Makes
4 eggs + 12 spears

Serving Size
2 eggs + 6 spears

INGREDIENTS

12 medium spears asparagus, tough ends trimmed

$1/4$ cup homemade chicken stock

2 tbsp animal fat (or ghee if dairy is tolerated)

2 tbsp chopped fresh basil, cilantro, mint, or Italian flat-leaf parsley

4 large eggs, pastured

$1/4$ tsp sea salt

METHOD

1 Place asparagus spears in an even layer in a medium skillet. Add chicken stock and animal fat, and sprinkle with herbs. Set heat to medium.

2 Crack 2 eggs over 6 asparagus spears and crack remaining 2 eggs over remaining 6 spears. Sprinkle sea salt evenly over eggs.

3 When stock begins to boil, cover, reduce heat to medium-low, and cook for 5 minutes or until egg whites are hardened and asparagus is just softened.

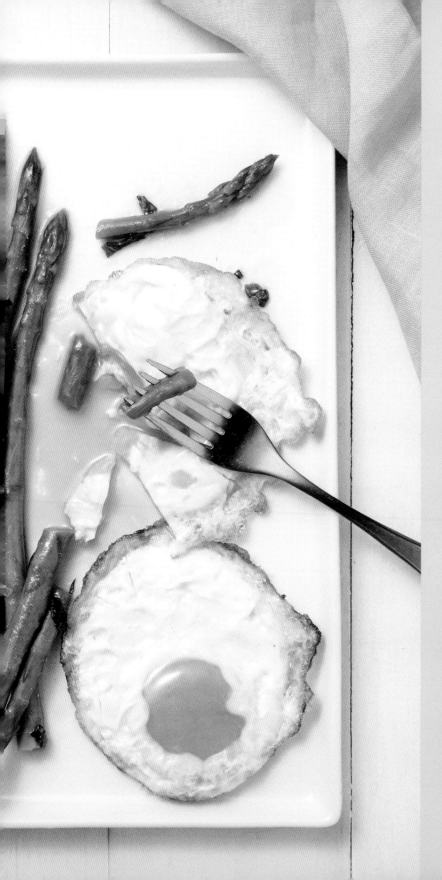

Variation

Grilled Steak and Asparagus with Poached Eggs

STAGE 4

INGREDIENTS
1 tsp ghee

½ tsp sea salt

12 medium asparagus spears

2 (6-oz; 170g) New York strip steaks

2 cups homemade chicken stock

4 large eggs

METHOD

1 Preheat the grill to medium. Spread ½ teaspoon ghee and ¼ teaspoon sea salt on asparagus. Cover both sides of New York strip steaks with remaining ½ teaspoon ghee and remaining ¼ teaspoon sea salt.

2 Grill steaks for 4 minutes per side, rotating 90 degrees halfway through the cook time. Flip over steaks and repeat. Add asparagus to the grill when you flip steaks, moving occasionally to cook evenly. Transfer steaks and asparagus to a plate, and let rest for 10 minutes.

3 In a medium saucepan over medium-high heat, bring chicken stock to a boil. Reduce heat to medium-low, gently crack eggs into stock, and simmer for 3 minutes or until whites are firm.

4 Divide steak, asparagus, and eggs between 2 plates. Season with sea salt, and serve.

Roasted Winter Squash Pancakes

These fluffy and delicate pancakes are a delight when served with sweet and nutty Almond Butter Honey Spread on top.

Prep Time
10 minutes

Cook Time
12 minutes

Makes
8 pancakes

Serving Size
2 pancakes

INGREDIENTS

2 cups roasted butternut or other winter squash purée, no skin or seeds

4 large egg yolks

$^3/_4$ tsp sea salt

$^1/_2$ cup ghee or animal fat

Almond Butter Honey Spread

METHOD

1 In a medium bowl, whisk together roasted winter squash, egg yolks, and sea salt.

2 Heat a large skillet over medium-low heat. Add $^1/_4$ cup ghee, and swirl the skillet to distribute.

3 Using a $^1/_4$-cup scoop, add squash mixture to the skillet. (You'll have to work in batches to avoid overcrowding the skillet.) Gently press down on each pancake with a spatula to flatten to $^1/_4$-inch (0.5cm) thickness. Cover, and cook pancakes for 3 minutes.

4 Uncover, flip over pancakes with spatula, re-cover, and cook for 3 more minutes.

5 Transfer cooked pancakes to a plate, and repeat with remaining squash mixture and remaining $^1/_4$ cup ghee. Serve topped with Almond Butter Honey Spread.

Topping

Almond Butter Honey Spread

STAGE 3

To make this delightful spread, whisk together $^1/_4$ cup all-natural almond butter and 4 teaspoons raw honey in a small bowl. Pour into a small pan, set over medium heat, and cook, whisking constantly, for 3 minutes. When honey and almond butter are combined and warmed, reduce heat to low.

Honey

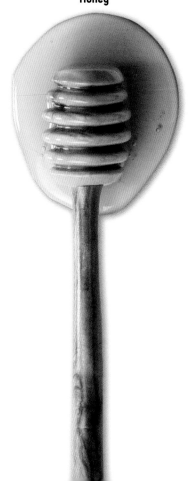

DAIRY FREE **NUT FREE** **PALEO DIET**

Easy Avocado Omelet

A fluffy, soft, and delicate blanket of eggs with smooth, rich avocado tucked in the center, this omelet is wonderful for any meal.

Prep Time
5 minutes

Cook Time
5 minutes

Makes
1 omelet

Serving Size
1 omelet

INGREDIENTS

2 large eggs

2 tbsp water

1/4 tsp sea salt

1 tbsp animal fat
(or ghee if dairy is
tolerated)

1/4 cup diced red onion

1/2 clove garlic, minced

1/4 cup mashed avocado

METHOD

1 In a small bowl, beat eggs, water, and sea salt until blended and foamy.

2 In a medium skillet or omelet pan over medium-high heat, heat animal fat. When hot, add red onion and garlic, and cook, stirring, for about 2 minutes.

3 Pour egg mixture in the center of the skillet. Using a spatula, gently push cooked parts of eggs from the outer edges of the skillet toward the center so uncooked eggs can reach hot skillet surface. Cook for about 2 minutes, gently moving cooked egg portions as needed until top surface of eggs is thickened and no visible liquid egg remains.

4 Place avocado on one side of cooked eggs, and use the spatula to fold omelet onto avocado.

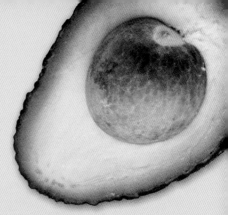

Avocado

Variation

Salmon, Spinach, and Tomato Omelet with Avocado

In addition to the ingredients in step 2, add 1/4 cup chopped red ripe tomato, 1/2 cup chopped baby spinach, and 1/4 cup poached and flaked salmon. After cooking 2 minutes, add 1 teaspoon fresh lemon juice and 2 teaspoons chopped fresh basil, and stir. Proceed with step 3.

STAGE 3

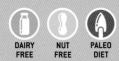

DAIRY FREE NUT FREE PALEO DIET

Aromatic Chicken with Mushrooms

Mushrooms, garlic, and onions make the perfect complement to this warm and filling dish. Serve with Simple Roasted Root Vegetables for a satisfying and gut-friendly meal.

Prep Time	**Cook Time**	**Makes**	**Serving Size**
15 minutes	30 minutes	4 chicken breasts	1 breast

INGREDIENTS

2 medium sweet or yellow onions, sliced thin

4 cups sliced button, cremini, or baby portobello mushrooms

2 cloves garlic, finely diced

2 tbsp coconut oil or lard (or ghee if dairy is tolerated)

4 (6-oz; 170g) skin-on chicken breasts

Sea salt

2 to 4 cups homemade chicken stock

METHOD

1 Preheat the oven to 350°F (180°C).

2 In a large ceramic casserole dish, combine sweet onions, button mushrooms, and garlic. Add coconut oil or lard, and place chicken breasts on top. Sprinkle with sea salt, and fill pan with chicken stock until just a bit of chicken skin is exposed.

3 Bake for 30 minutes or until chicken skin is brown and slightly crispy.

4 To serve, top chicken breasts with mushrooms and onions.

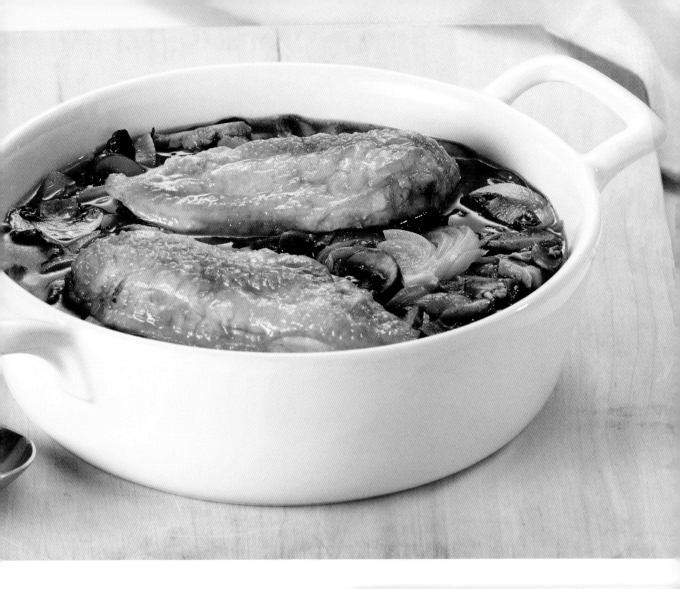

Side Dish

Simple Roasted Root Vegetables

Chop 1 medium beet, 3 large carrots, and 2 medium turnips into 1/2-inch (1.25cm) dice. Toss with 2 tablespoons melted coconut oil and 1/2 teaspoon sea salt, and place in a 9×13-inch (23×33cm) baking dish. Bake at 400°F (200°C) for 45 minutes, tossing once at 20 minutes. (Makes 4 servings.)

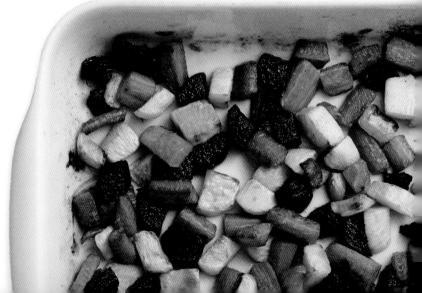

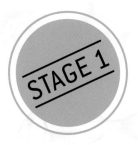

STAGE 1

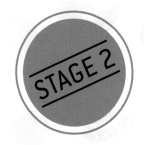

STAGE 2

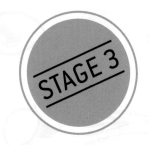

STAGE 3

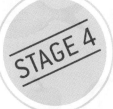

STAGE 4

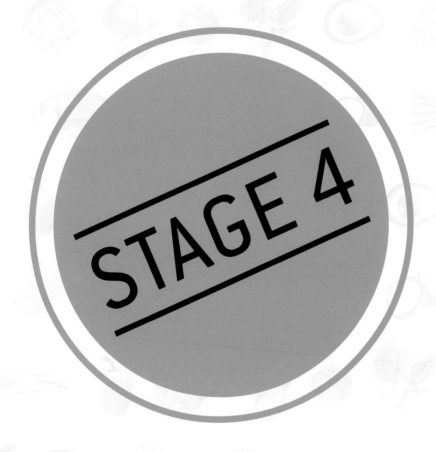

STAGE 4

STAGE 5

STAGE 6

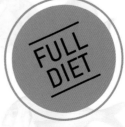

FULL
DIET

DAIRY FREE

PALEO DIET

Ginger Pumpkin Muffins

The deeply rich flavor of pumpkin spice is baked into a delicate, soft, and satisfying muffin that's great any time of year.

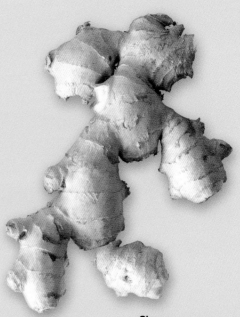

Ginger

Prep Time	Cook Time	Makes	Serving Size
15 minutes	25 minutes	12 muffins	1 muffin

INGREDIENTS

3 cups almond flour

½ tsp baking soda

¼ tsp sea salt

1½ tsp ground cinnamon

1½ tsp ground ginger

¼ tsp ground nutmeg

¼ cup walnut pieces, soaked and dried

1 cup canned, unsweetened pumpkin purée, or homemade roasted pumpkin/winter squash purée

¼ cup raw honey

4 large pastured eggs

½ tsp pure vanilla extract

METHOD

1 Preheat the oven to 325°F (170°C). Oil the bottoms and sides of 3×2-inch (7.5×6.25cm) nonstick muffin pan cups with 1 teaspoon coconut oil.

2 In a medium bowl, combine almond flour, baking soda, sea salt, cinnamon, ginger, nutmeg, and walnuts.

3 In a separate medium bowl, whisk together pumpkin purée, honey, eggs, and vanilla extract.

4 Pour dry ingredients into wet ingredients, and stir until well combined.

5 Fill each muffin cup with ¼ cup batter, and bake on the middle oven rack for 25 minutes or until a toothpick inserted into middle of muffin comes out clean.

6 Cool muffins for 15 minutes before serving. Remove cooled muffins from the muffin tin using a rubber spatula if needed.

DAIRY FREE

PALEO DIET

Chicken Muffins

Cook a double or triple batch of these protein-packed muffins on the weekend, freeze, and you'll have quick and easy meals or snacks throughout the busy week to reheat and enjoy.

Prep Time	Cook Time	Makes	Serving Size
20 minutes	35 minutes	6 muffins	1 muffins

INGREDIENTS

$1/4$ cup diced yellow onion

$1/4$ cup chopped green bell pepper

$1/4$ cup peeled and chopped carrot

$1/4$ cup chopped yellow squash

2 cloves garlic, minced

$1^1/2$ lb (680g) ground chicken, preferably dark meat

$1/2$ tsp sea salt

$1/4$ tsp ground black pepper

$1/4$ tsp dried oregano

$1/4$ tsp dried basil

$1/4$ tsp dried rosemary

1 large egg

$1/2$ cup almond flour

2 tbsp sugar-free tomato paste

METHOD

1 Preheat the oven to 350°F (180°C). Lightly oil a 6-cup king-size (3.5×3-inch; 9×7.5cm) muffin tin with animal fat or coconut oil.

2 In a medium skillet over medium-high heat, sauté yellow onion, green bell pepper, carrot, yellow squash, and garlic for 3 or 4 minutes or until soft. Set aside to cool.

3 In a large bowl, and using clean hands, combine chicken, sautéed vegetables, sea salt, black pepper, oregano, basil, rosemary, egg, almond flour, and tomato paste.

4 Divide chicken mixture evenly among the 6 muffin cups, and bake for 35 minutes.

5 Serve immediately, or freeze muffins individually.

To make these low FODMAP, omit the onion and garlic.

Yellow squash

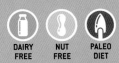

DAIRY FREE   **NUT FREE**   **PALEO DIET**

Green Goddess Juice

This refreshing elixir is full of antioxidants, minerals, and compounds that supercharge the liver, help digestion, and lower inflammation.

Prep Time
15 minutes

Makes
2 cups

Serving Size
1 cup

INGREDIENTS

1 cup baby spinach
1 cup kale, thick ends trimmed
$\frac{1}{2}$ cup peeled, seeded, and chopped cucumber
1 small green apple, cored
Juice of $\frac{1}{2}$ small lime
$\frac{1}{4}$ cup fresh cilantro leaves
1 medium kiwifruit, peeled
1 tbsp fresh ginger

METHOD

1 Process baby spinach, kale, cucumber, green apple, lime juice, cilantro, kiwifruit, and ginger through a juicer, or purée in a blender. If blending, strain into a small bowl by squeezing pulp through four layers of cheesecloth.

2 Serve juice immediately.

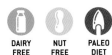

DAIRY FREE   **NUT FREE**   **PALEO DIET**

Peppery Pear Juice

Peppery arugula is mellowed by the sweetness of pears in this tasty juice. Lemon adds a pop of citrus and helps cleanse the liver.

Prep Time
15 minutes

Makes
2 cups

Serving Size
1 cup

INGREDIENTS

4 medium pears, cored, seeded, and quartered
1 medium lemon, seeded and white pith removed
4 large stalks celery
3 cups arugula

METHOD

1 Process pears, lemon, celery, and arugula through a juicer, or purée in a blender. If blending, strain into a small bowl by squeezing pulp through four layers of cheesecloth.

2 Serve juice immediately.

> These juices help keep the liver healthy so it can keep processing the high-quality fats you're consuming to heal your gut.

DAIRY FREE **NUT FREE** **PALEO DIET**

Liver-Loving Juice

Beets and ginger pack a powerful punch. Beets help keep your liver healthy and producing bile to digest gut-healing high-quality fat. Ginger calms your stomach and helps boost your immune system.

Prep Time
15 minutes

Makes
2 cups

Serving Size
1 cup

INGREDIENTS

- 1 (1½-in; 3.75cm) piece ginger, peeled and chopped
- 4 large carrots, peeled and coarsely chopped
- 1 large beet, scrubbed and cut into 2-in (5cm) chunks
- 1 medium Honeycrisp or Gala apple, cored and cut into eighths

METHOD

1 Process ginger, carrots, beet, and Honeycrisp apple through a juicer, or purée in a blender. If blending, strain into a small bowl by squeezing pulp through four layers of cheesecloth.

2 Serve juice immediately.

Variation

Golden Goddess Juice

Replace the medium apple with a medium orange, peeled, seeded, and white pith removed. Reduce the carrots to 2, and add 3 cups spinach.

STAGE 4

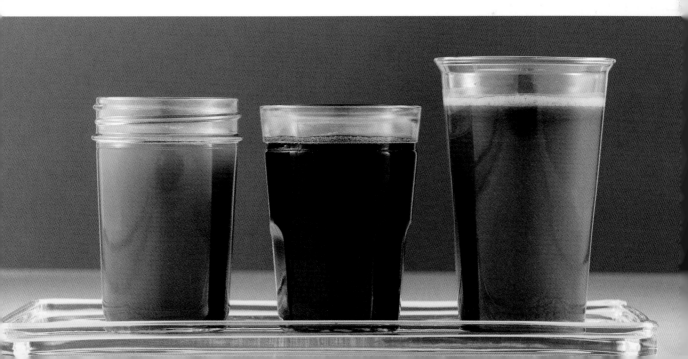

DAIRY FREE

NUT FREE

PALEO DIET

Garlic Chicken with Vegetables

Buttery-sweet garlic-crisped skin accompanies delicious, moist chicken in this one-pot dish. Juices from the chicken help create caramelized, tender vegetables. You can easily change the veggies to meet your preference and stage.

Prep Time
15 minutes

Cook Time
60 minutes

Makes
4 cups + 8 thighs

Serving Size
1 cup + 2 thighs

INGREDIENTS

1 cup halved and then quartered yellow onion

1 cup carrots, peeled and cut into 1-in (2.5cm) rounds

1 cup celery, cut into 2-in (5cm) pieces

1 cup fresh whole green beans, ends trimmed, and halved crosswise

3 tbsp animal fat (or ghee if dairy is tolerated)

2 tsp rosemary

1 tbsp sea salt

8 bone-in, skin-on chicken thighs (about 3 lb; 1.5kg)

4 cloves garlic

2 tbsp chopped fresh thyme

METHOD

1 Preheat the oven to 400°F (205°C).

2 In a large bowl, combine vegetables, 1 tablespoon animal fat, rosemary, and 1 teaspoon sea salt. Transfer to an ovenproof glass baking dish, and spread into an even layer.

3 In the same bowl, toss together chicken, remaining 2 teaspoons sea salt, garlic, thyme, and remaining 2 tablespoons animal fat.

4 Evenly distribute thighs in dish, evenly distributed over vegetables. Bake on middle oven rack for 60 minutes or until it reaches 165°F (75°C).

Q&A

What's the best way to store herbs?

Herbs are often sold in bundles larger than what you might need for a recipe. Rather than throw away the extra herbs or let them spoil before you're able to use them, learn how easy it is to properly store them for later use. For delicate herbs like Italian flat-leaf parsley, basil, and mint, trim off the ends and discard any browned leaves. Add 1 inch (2.5cm) water to a glass jar, place the herbs trimmed side down in the jar, cover with the lid or a plastic bag, and refrigerate. For hardier herbs like thyme and rosemary, place the herbs in a single layer on a moist paper towel, roll up the towel, and refrigerate the wrapped herbs in a zipper-lock plastic bag. Change the paper towel or jar water weekly.

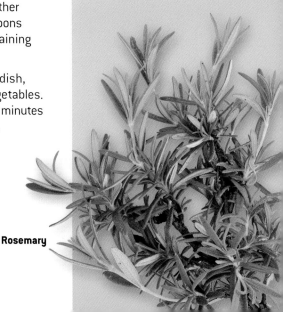
Rosemary

Grilled Salmon with Walnut Pesto

The perfect balance of fresh herbs and zesty lemon brings a wonderful brightness to slightly smoky, omega-3-rich grilled salmon.

Prep Time
10 minutes

Cook Time
10 minutes

Makes
4 fillets + 1½ cups pesto

Serving Size
1 fillet + 2 tablespoons pesto

INGREDIENTS

½ tsp sea salt

3 cloves garlic

1 cup walnuts, soaked and dried

1 cup fresh Italian flat-leaf parsley

2 tbsp fresh chives

2 tbsp fresh cilantro leaves

2 tbsp fresh basil leaves

3 tsp grated lemon zest

½ cup virgin olive oil

1½ lb (680g) wild salmon, cut into 4 (6-oz; 170g) fillets

METHOD

1 Preheat the grill to medium.

2 In a food processor fitted with a metal chopping blade, process sea salt, garlic, walnuts, Italian flat-leaf parsley, chives, cilantro, basil, lemon zest, and virgin olive oil until smooth.

3 Place salmon skin side up on the grill, close the lid, and cook for 5 minutes, rotating fish 90 degrees halfway through the cook time.

4 Flip over fish, spread 2 tablespoons pesto on the grill-marked side of each salmon fillet, close the lid, and cook 5 more minutes, rotating fish 90 degrees halfway through cook time.

Q&A

What can I do with leftover pesto?

You'll have 1 cup leftover pesto with this recipe. You can use it as a condiment for grilled chicken or roast beef, mix it in with scrambled eggs, or serve as a dip for vegetables. Or for a quick and easy bruschetta, spread some pesto on a piece of toasted Everyday Grain-Free Bread, top with chopped red ripe tomatoes and a little sea salt, and enjoy! Just remember to refrigerate the extra pesto tightly covered until ready to use.

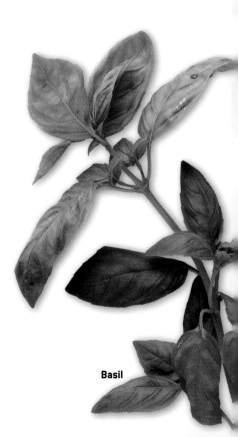

Basil

NUT FREE

"Noodles" with Pomodoro Sauce

These long, soft, delicate zucchini noodles will curb any pasta craving—especially when paired with your choice of sauce. This sauce is a light tomato and basil pomodoro, but the options are endless.

Prep Time	**Cook Time**	**Makes**	**Serving Size**
15 minutes	5 minutes	4 cups	2 cups

INGREDIENTS

2 medium zucchini or summer squashes, ends trimmed

$1^1/_2$ cups diced tomatoes

$^1/_2$ cup chopped fresh basil leaves

1 clove garlic, chopped

$^1/_4$ tsp sea salt

$^1/_4$ tsp black pepper

2 tbsp ghee

METHOD

1 Lay a box grater flat on your workstation so the largest holes face up. Push zucchini longwise across the top of the grater, rotate zucchini, and push across the grater again. Repeat until all zucchini is shredded into noodles. (Or use a vegetable spiralizer or mandoline slicer.)

2 In a medium bowl, combine tomatoes, basil, garlic, sea salt, and black pepper.

3 In a medium skillet over medium heat, heat ghee. Add 4 cups zucchini noodles, and cook, stirring occasionally, for $3^1/_2$ minutes or until just softened.

4 Add 2 cups sauce to noodles, and cook, stirring to warm sauce and completely coat noodles, for $1^1/_2$ minutes.

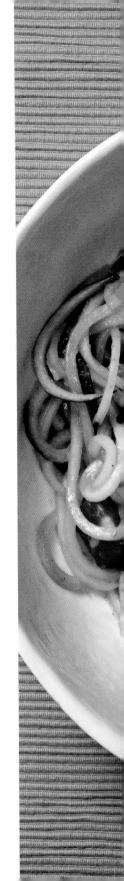

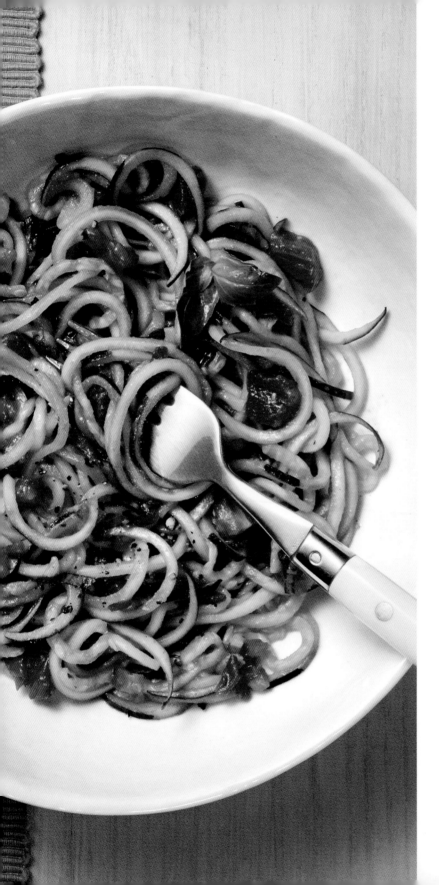

Variations

Tahini Lemon Sauce

STAGE 4

In a food processor or blender, chop 4 whole scallions, $1/4$ cup fresh cilantro leaves, 1 tablespoon crushed red pepper flakes (optional), 2 teaspoons sesame seeds, $1/4$ cup tahini, $1/4$ cup lemon juice, 2 teaspoons sesame oil, 1 teaspoon honey, $1/4$ cup stock, $1/2$ teaspoon sea salt, and $1/4$ teaspoon black pepper until smooth.

Spinach Pesto Sauce

FULL DIET

In a food processor or blender, chop $1/2$ cup soaked and dried walnuts, 2 cups fresh Italian flat-leaf parsley, 2 cups baby spinach, 2 cloves garlic, $1/2$ cup cut chives, $1/4$ teaspoon sea salt, and $1/4$ teaspoon black pepper. With the food processor on low speed, slowly drizzle in $3/4$ cup virgin olive oil. When combined, stir in $1/2$ cup grated Parmesan cheese.

DAIRY FREE   PALEO DIET

Oven-Roasted Turkey Meatloaf

This fresh and filling meatloaf is moist, juicy, and delicious—and the vegetables are cooked right in. For a quick meal, place a slice of leftover meatloaf between two slices of Everyday Grain-Free Bread, and enjoy!

Prep Time	**Cook Time**	**Makes**	**Serving Size**
15 minutes	60 minutes	8 (1-inch; 2.5cm) slices	1 slice

INGREDIENTS

3/4 cup diced yellow onion

1 cup tomato purée

2 tbsp raw honey

2 lb (1kg) ground turkey

2 large eggs, beaten

1/2 cup almond meal

1 cup chopped frozen spinach, thawed, squeezed, and drained

2 cloves garlic, minced

1/2 cup diced scallions, green part only

1/2 cup diced red bell pepper

1/2 cup peeled and grated carrot

1/2 cup sliced shiitake mushroom caps

1 tsp sea salt

METHOD

1 Preheat the oven to 350ºF (180ºC). In a small bowl, whisk together 1/4 cup yellow onion, tomato purée, and honey.

2 In a medium bowl, combine turkey, eggs, almond meal, remaining 1/2 cup yellow onion, spinach, garlic, scallions, red bell pepper, carrot, shiitake mushrooms, and sea salt. Transfer mixture to a 9×13-inch (23×33cm) ovenproof baking dish, and using your hands, form into a 6×3-inch (15.25×7.5cm) loaf.

3 Pour tomato purée mixture evenly over meatloaf, and spread to evenly coat sides and top.

4 Bake on the middle oven rack for 60 minutes or until internal temperature reaches 160ºF (70ºC). Cool meatloaf for 10 minutes before slicing and serving.

If turkey isn't your preference, substitute 2 pounds (1kg) ground chicken or beef. Prepare as directed. Or combine equal portions chicken, turkey, and beef.

DAIRY FREE **NUT FREE** **PALEO DIET**

Classic Pot Roast with Onions

Lightly seasoned beef is slow roasted and braised in its own juices with fresh, aromatic garlic and onions and hearty rosemary and thyme.

Prep Time	**Cook Time**	**Makes**	**Serving Size**
15 minutes	4 hours	1 roast	¹/₈ of roast

INGREDIENTS

¹/₂ tsp sea salt

1 (4-lb; 2kg) beef chuck roast

2 tbsp animal fat (or ghee if dairy is tolerated)

4 medium yellow onions, quartered

4 medium carrots, peeled and cut into 2-in (5cm) pieces

4 cloves garlic, halved

3 sprigs rosemary

5 sprigs thyme

3 cups homemade beef stock

METHOD

1 Preheat the oven to 275ºF (140ºC). Spread sea salt evenly on all sides of chuck roast.

2 In a large ovenproof stockpot or Dutch oven over medium heat, heat 1 tablespoon animal fat. Add yellow onions, carrots, garlic, rosemary, and thyme, and sauté, stirring, for 4 minutes or until lightly browned. Carefully transfer to a plate.

3 Add remaining 1 tablespoon animal fat to the pot, add roast, and sear for 1 minute per side or until browned. Turn off heat, and transfer roast to a plate.

4 Return vegetables and herbs to the pot, lay roast on top of vegetables and herbs, and add beef stock. Cover pot, and cook on the middle oven rack for 4 hours or until tender.

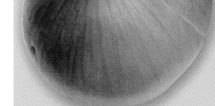

Yellow onions

Variation

Slow Cooker Pot Roast with Onions

STAGE 4

Omit the fat, and combine the sea salt, carrots, garlic, yellow onions, rosemary and thyme tied with butchers twine or cheesecloth for easy removal, and beef stock in a 6-quart (5.5-liter) slow cooker. Add the roast, cover, and cook on low for 8 hours. Carefully remove the roast and allow to sit for 5 minutes before slicing it against the grain.

NUT FREE

Ground Beef Stroganoff

Tender beef and mushrooms pair with a tangy homemade yogurt sauce. So delicious and simple, this quick and easy recipe is sure to become your go-to meal on busy weeknights, especially when served with Butternut Squash Gnocchi.

Prep Time
10 minutes

Cook Time
25 minutes

Makes
4 cups

Serving Size
1 cup

INGREDIENTS

- 1 lb (450g) ground beef
- 2 cups sliced brown button mushrooms
- 1 cup chopped yellow onion
- 3 cloves garlic, chopped
- 1 1/3 cups homemade beef stock
- 1/2 tsp sea salt
- 1 tsp chopped fresh rosemary
- 1/4 cup chopped fresh parsley
- 1 cup homemade yogurt
- 1/4 cup ghee or animal fat

METHOD

1 In a large skillet, combine ground beef, brown button mushrooms, yellow onion, garlic, beef stock, and sea salt. Set heat to medium-high heat, and bring to a boil.

2 Cover, reduce heat to medium-low, and cook for 20 minutes. Turn off heat.

3 Fold in rosemary and parsley. Serve topped with a dollop of homemade yogurt and a drizzle of ghee.

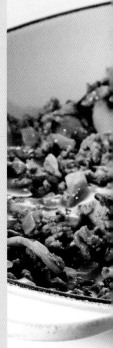

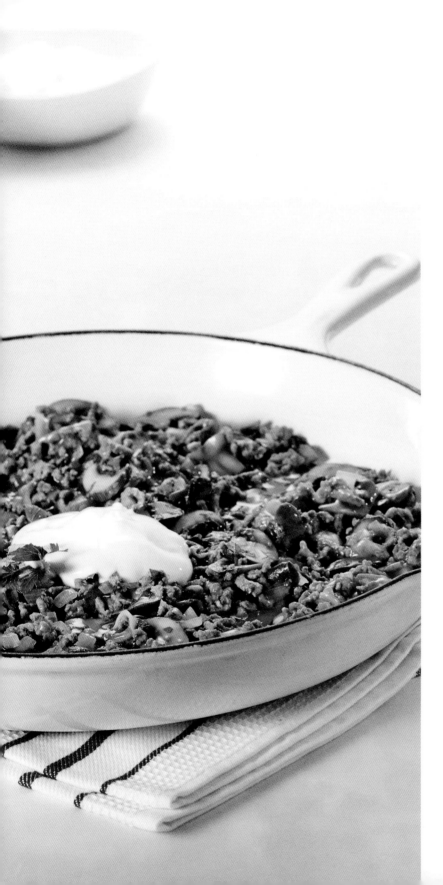

Side Dish

Butternut Squash Gnocchi

FULL DIET

INGREDIENTS
1 large egg
1 cup mashed butternut squash
1½ cups almond flour
¼ cup coconut flour
¼ cup grated Parmesan cheese
1½ tsp sea salt
½ tsp black pepper
¼ tsp ground nutmeg

METHOD
1 In a medium bowl, gently whisk egg until yolk and white are combined. Add butternut squash, almond flour, coconut flour, Parmesan cheese, sea salt, black pepper, and nutmeg, and mix well.

2 Form the dough into a tight mound. Scoop out 1 tablespoon, roll between palms to form a small ball, and squeeze gently between your thumb and index finger to form a small cylinder. Gently drag the tines of a fork over top. Repeat.

3 Fill a medium saucepan with enough water to cover the bottom 2 inches (5cm), set over medium-high heat, bring to a boil, and reduce heat to a simmer.

4 Add 10 gnocchi at a time, and cook for 2 minutes. Using a slotted spoon, transfer gnocchi to plate to drain, and repeat with remaining gnocchi.

DAIRY FREE   **PALEO DIET**

Ground Beef Empanadas

The nuttiness of almond flour, citrus-toned cilantro, and tangy lime combine to give these savory stuffed and baked pastry pillows an island feel. They're just the right size for an afternoon snack!

Prep Time	Cook Time	Makes	Serving Size
15 minutes	30 minutes	14 empanadas	2 empanadas

INGREDIENTS

4 cups almond flour

4 large pastured eggs

8 tbsp coconut oil, melted over low heat

3 tsp sea salt

3 tbsp animal fat (or ghee if dairy is tolerated)

1^1/$_2$ lb (680g) ground beef

6 cloves garlic, minced

1^1/$_2$ cups diced yellow onion

2^1/$_4$ cups chopped red ripe tomatoes

^{1}/$_3$ cup tomato purée

^{1}/$_3$ cup beef stock

^{1}/$_3$ cup fresh cilantro leaves

1 tbsp fresh lime juice

METHOD

1 Preheat the oven to 350°F (180°C). Line a baking sheet with parchment paper.

2 In a medium bowl, combine almond flour, eggs, coconut oil, and 1^1/$_2$ teaspoons sea salt. Form and press dough into a mound, wrap in plastic wrap, and refrigerate until needed.

3 In a medium skillet over medium heat, combine animal fat, ground beef, garlic, remaining 1^1/$_2$ teaspoons sea salt, and yellow onion, and cook, stirring and breaking up larger chunks, for 5 minutes.

4 Add tomatoes, tomato purée, and beef stock, and cook for 10 minutes or until beef is fully cooked and liquid is mostly reduced. Add cilantro and lime juice, stir to combine, and set aside to cool completely.

5 Divide dough into 14 (small, ^{1}/$_4$ cup) mounds. Place a 6×6-inch (15.25×15.25cm) piece parchment paper or plastic wrap on your counter. Set 1 dough ball on parchment paper, and flatten it to a 4- or 5-inch (10 or 12.5cm) circle. Place 3 tablespoons cooled ground beef mixture on half of dough circle, carefully lift opposite side of parchment paper, fold it over to enclose beef mixture, and press gently to seal. (Note dough doesn't contain gluten so it won't be stretchy.) Repeat with remaining dough and beef mixture.

6 Gently place formed empanadas on the baking sheet using a spatula. Bake on the middle oven rack for 20 minutes or until dough is browned and beef filling is warmed.

DAIRY FREE

PALEO DIET

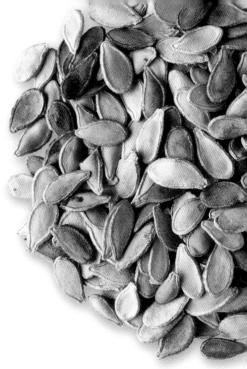

Crackling Nuts

Nuts contain phytic acid, which binds to minerals during digestion and prevents the body from properly absorbing them. Soaking nuts in saltwater neutralizes the phytic acid, making the nuts easier to digest.

Prep Time	Cook Time	Makes	Serving Size
5 minutes	12 to 24 hours	4 cups	$1/4$ cup

INGREDIENTS

4 cups pecans, walnuts, pine nuts, macadamia nuts, hazelnuts, or cashews

Warm spring or filtered water

1 tbsp sea salt

METHOD

1 Place nuts in a medium bowl, add warm spring water to cover, season with sea salt, and stir to combine. Set aside at room temperature for 7 hours.

2 Strain nuts through a fine-mesh strainer, and rinse. Spread in an even layer on a baking sheet and bake for 12 to 24 hours at no more than 150°F (65°C). (Or use a dehydrator.)

3 Refrigerate nuts in an airtight container for up to 3 months, or freeze for up to 6 months.

Variation

Crackling Seeds

STAGE 4

Swap out the nuts for your favorite seeds. Seeds such as sunflower and pumpkin seeds also contain phytic acid and should be soaked and dried as directed.

To make this recipe low FODMAP, do not use cashews (or pistachios).

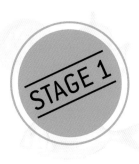

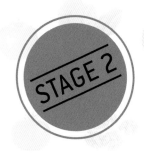

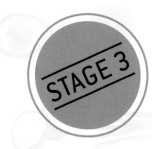

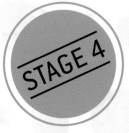

STAGE 5

STAGE 5

STAGE 6

FULL
DIET

DAIRY FREE **NUT FREE** **LOW FODMAP** **PALEO DIET**

Simple House Salad

Now that you can tolerate raw vegetables, you can easily increase your intake with this quick combination of tender lettuces and refreshing cucumbers in a tangy and fruity vinaigrette.

Prep Time
10 minutes

Makes
2 salads

Serving Size
1 salad

INGREDIENTS

1 tbsp fresh lemon juice

3 tbsp virgin olive oil

$1/2$ tsp sea salt

4 cups chopped butter lettuce, soft leaves

1 cup cucumber, peeled, seeded, and sliced into thin rounds

METHOD

1 In a small bowl, whisk together lemon juice, virgin olive oil, and sea salt.

2 Place butter lettuce and cucumber in a medium bowl, pour lemon vinaigrette over top, and toss to coat.

In addition to soft butter lettuce, red leaf, baby spinach, and romaine work well in this recipe.

Variation

Garden Salad

STAGE 5

Add $1/2$ cup peeled and shredded carrot, $1/2$ cup chopped or sliced red ripe tomato, and 1 slice red Bermuda onion. In stage 6, you can incorporate $1/2$ cup raw fruit such as apples, berries, cherries, and grapes.

Butter lettuce

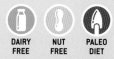

DAIRY FREE **NUT FREE** **PALEO DIET**

Grain-Free Tabbouleh

In this updated version of the traditional Lebanese salad, parsley adds good-for-you minerals and antioxidants. Substitute cauliflower for the usual bulgur for an interesting variation.

Prep Time
20 minutes

Cook Time
5 minutes

Makes
8 to 10 cups

Serving Size
1/3 cup

INGREDIENTS

- 1/2 head cauliflower, florets only, chopped extremely finely with a knife or in a food processor
- 3 bunches fresh Italian flat-leaf parsley, finely chopped (about 2 cups)
- 1/2 cup finely chopped fresh mint
- 2 medium tomatoes, cut into 1/4-in (0.5cm) dice
- 1/2 medium cucumber, peeled, cored, seeded, and cut into 1/4-in (0.5cm) dice
- 3 tbsp olive oil
- 3 tbsp fresh lemon juice
- 3/4 tsp sea salt
- 1/4 tsp black pepper

METHOD

1 In a small saucepan over high heat, bring 3 cups water to a boil. Reduce heat to medium-low, add cauliflower, and cook for 5 minutes.

2 Drain cauliflower in a fine-mesh strainer and transfer to a medium bowl.

3 Add Italian flat-leaf parsley, mint, tomatoes, cucumber, olive oil, lemon juice, sea salt, and black pepper, and mix well until combined. Serve immediately or refrigerate tightly covered for up to 1 week.

After stage 2, consider roasting the cauliflower instead of boiling it. Toss finely diced or processed cauliflower with coconut oil or animal fat, season with 1 teaspoon sea salt, and roast on a baking sheet at 425°F (220°C) for 25 to 40 minutes, depending on how brown and crispy you want it.

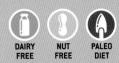

DAIRY FREE **NUT FREE** **PALEO DIET**

Mini Butternut Squash Soufflés

Light, fluffy, and subtly sweet, these easy butternut squash soufflés are a great option for weekend brunches.

Prep Time
10 minutes

Cook Time
30 minutes

Makes
6 soufflés

Serving Size
1 soufflé

INGREDIENTS

12 large pastured eggs

1$\frac{1}{2}$ cups butternut squash purée

1 tsp sea salt

Raw honey (optional)

METHOD

1 Preheat the oven to 350°F (180°C). Grease 6 (2-cup) ramekins with coconut oil.

2 In a medium bowl, whisk eggs until beaten. Add butternut squash purée and sea salt, mix well, and pour into the prepared ramekins.

3 Bake for 30 minutes or until soufflés have puffed up and a skewer or knife inserted into the center of one comes out clean.

4 Drizzle soufflés with raw honey (if using), and serve.

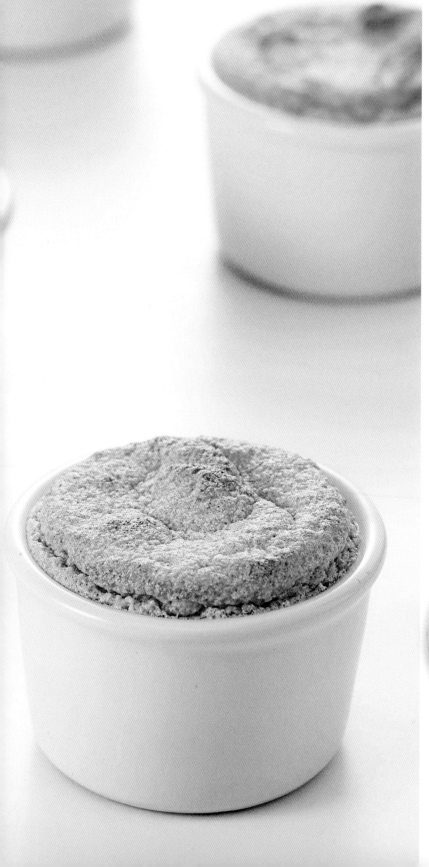

Component

Butternut Squash Purée

To make your own butternut squash purée, follow these steps:

1 Preheat the oven to 400°F (200°C). Cut 1 medium butternut squash in half, and remove the seeds.

2 Place on a baking sheet, and roast for 45 minutes or until soft and easily pierced with a fork.

3 Scoop squash into a blender or a food processor fitted with a metal chopping blade, and process until smooth. (You might need to do this in batches.)

4 Refrigerate for up to 1 week.

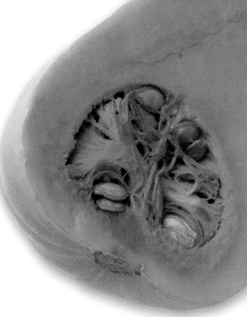

Butternut squash

DAIRY FREE **NUT FREE** **PALEO DIET**

Guacamole

The smooth, creamy texture of avocados makes this guacamole a hit. The bright green flesh creates a pop of color, and the healthy fat nourishes your body. Serve with sliced vegetables for an even healthier option.

Prep Time	Makes	Serving Size
15 minutes	2 or 3 cups	$^1/_4$ cup

INGREDIENTS

3 medium avocados
$^1/_2$ large tomato, diced
$^1/_2$ medium red onion, diced
2 cloves garlic, minced
Juice of 1 small lime
$^1/_2$ tsp sea salt, or to taste
$^1/_4$ tsp black pepper
$^1/_4$ tsp turmeric

METHOD

1 Split avocados, and remove pits. Scoop flesh into a medium bowl, and mash with a fork until smooth with some small chunks.

2 Add tomato, red onion, garlic, lime juice, sea salt, black pepper, and turmeric, and mix with a spatula until combined.

3 Serve immediately, or refrigerate in an airtight container for up to 6 hours.

Variations

Sun-Dried Tomato Guacamole

FULL DIET

Omit the lime juice and turmeric, and replace the tomato with 15 sun-dried tomatoes, rehydrated and chopped. Replace the red onion with $^1/_2$ cup hearts of palm, diced. Add 2 tablespoons grated Romano cheese and 1 tablespoon capers. Continue as directed.

Pesto Guacamole

STAGE 4

Omit the lime juice and turmeric, and replace the tomato with 30 medium or large basil leaves, cut into ribbons. Replace the red onion with 2 tablespoons pine nuts, soaked in water overnight. Continue as directed.

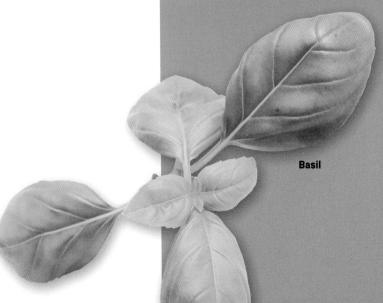

Basil

DAIRY FREE · **NUT FREE** · **PALEO DIET**

Easy Chicken Stir-Fry

This stir-fry is simple, quick, and satisfying. It's a great way to use leftover chicken and vegetables, too.

Prep Time	Cook Time	Makes	Serving Size
10 minutes	20 minutes	4 cups	1 cup

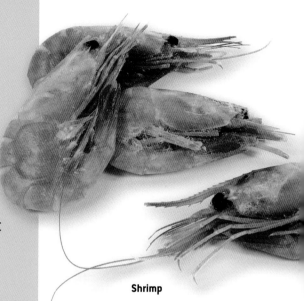

Shrimp

INGREDIENTS

- 2 tbsp coconut oil or animal fat
- 1 medium yellow onion, chopped
- 1 clove garlic, minced
- 1 lb (450g) chicken meat, preferably dark, sliced into strips
- 1 tsp sea salt
- 1 tsp ground black pepper
- 2 cups broccoli florets
- 1 medium carrot, peeled and shredded
- Juice of 1 small lime
- 4 tbsp shredded, unsweetened coconut
- Coconut aminos

METHOD

1 In a medium skillet over medium-high heat, melt coconut oil. Add yellow onion, and sauté for 5 minutes or until translucent.

2 Add garlic, and sauté for 3 minutes or until fragrant.

3 Season chicken with $^1/_2$ teaspoon sea salt and $^1/_2$ teaspoon black pepper. Add chicken to the skillet, and cook for 7 to 10 minutes or until no longer pink in center.

4 Add broccoli, carrot, and lime juice; sprinkle with remaining $^1/_2$ teaspoon sea salt and remaining $^1/_2$ teaspoon black pepper; and cook for 5 minutes.

5 To serve, sprinkle 1 tablespoon coconut sprinkled over each serving and top with coconut aminos to taste.

Variation

Spicy Shrimp Stir-Fry

STAGE 5

Use 1 pound (450g) shrimp instead of the chicken. For the vegetables, sauté onions and garlic as directed, and use 1 cup bok choy, 1 cup cabbage, and 1 cup pea pods instead of broccoli and carrots. Use lime juice and add $^1/_4$ teaspoon coriander, $^1/_4$ teaspoon ground ginger, and 1 pinch red chile flakes (optional). Sprinkle with diced cashews instead of flaked coconut and coconut aminos.

To make this dish low FODMAP, omit the onion, garlic, and coconut aminos (or use less than ¼ teaspoon of the latter).

DAIRY FREE

PALEO DIET

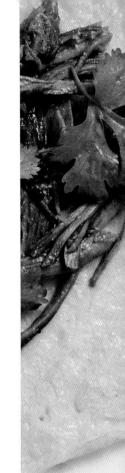

Tex-Mex Pulled Pork Burritos

In this dish, tender, slow-cooked pork is blanketed in a soft wrap and smothered with mildly spiced Tex-Mex-style sauce.

Prep Time
15 minutes

Cook Time
15 minutes

Makes
8 burritos + 4 cups sauce

Serving Size
1 burrito + 1/2 cup sauce

INGREDIENTS

2 tbsp sea salt

1 tsp black pepper

2 tsp paprika

1/2 tsp dry mustard powder

1 1/2 tsp ground cumin

1/2 tsp chipotle powder

8 lb (4kg) bone-in Boston butt pork shoulder

2 tbsp animal fat (or ghee if dairy is tolerated)

3 cups homemade chicken stock

1 cup chopped yellow onion

3 cloves garlic, chopped

2 tsp chili powder

3 cups tomato purée

1 cup apple cider vinegar

1 tsp ground cumin

1/2 cup raw honey

1/4 cup fresh cilantro leaves

8 Almond Flour Wraps

METHOD

1 Preheat the oven to 325°F (170°C). In a small bowl, combine sea salt, black pepper, paprika, dry mustard powder, cumin, and chipotle powder. Rub Boston butt pork shoulder completely with spice mixture.

2 Heat a large stockpot over medium-high heat, and add animal fat. Add pork shoulder, and cook, turning occasionally, for 6 minutes or until lightly browned on all sides.

3 Position pork fat side up and add 2 cups chicken stock, yellow onion, and garlic. Cover, and bake for 4 hours or until meat shreds easily with a fork. Remove from the oven, allow to cool completely, and pull pork from the bone.

4 Place the pot over medium-high heat, bring to a boil, and reduce heat to medium-low. Add chili powder, tomato purée, apple cider vinegar, remaining 1 cup chicken stock, cumin, honey, and cilantro, and cook uncovered for 20 minutes or until sauce is reduced to 4 cups. Working in small batches, blend sauce in a blender until smooth.

5 To serve, place 1/2 cup pulled pork in the center of 1 Almond Flour Wrap, fold in edges of wrap, and roll wrap to close, starting with edge closest to you. Smother burritos with sauce.

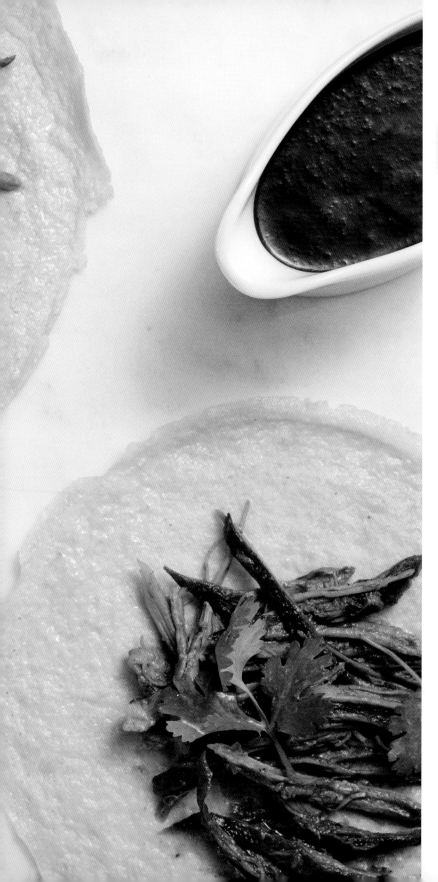

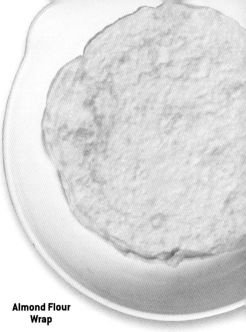

Almond Flour Wrap

Component

Almond Flour Wraps

STAGE 4

INGREDIENTS

5 large pastured eggs
3 tbsp water
¼ tsp sea salt
½ cup almond flour
Ghee, for brushing

METHOD

1 In a medium bowl, whisk together eggs, water, and sea salt. Slowly whisk in almond flour until batter is smooth and combined. Cover and refrigerate 10 minutes to allow batter to thicken.

2 Heat a large skillet over medium heat, brush with ghee, add ¼ cup batter, and swirl the skillet to coat with batter.

3 Cook for 1 minute or until wrap is set and firm to the touch. Using a spatula, carefully flip over wrap, and cook for 30 seconds. Transfer wrap to a plate, and repeat with remaining batter.

DAIRY FREE

NUT FREE

PALEO DIET

Apple Pie Stewed Apples

Nothing beats the warm, fall-spiced flavors of apple pie. These thinly sliced, softened jewels are great all on their own, even without the crust. Better yet, pair them with pork or winter squash pancakes.

Prep Time	Cook Time	Makes	Serving Size
10 minutes	30 minutes	3 cups	½ cup

INGREDIENTS

9 cups sweet red apples (about 3 lb; 1.5kg) such as Macintosh, Rome, Gala, or Honeycrisp, cored, peeled, and sliced into ¼-in (0.5cm) slices

2 tbsp water

2 tbsp animal fat (or ghee if dairy is tolerated)

½ tsp ground cinnamon

1 tsp ground allspice

½ tsp ground nutmeg

½ tsp ground ginger

¼ tsp ground cloves

⅛ tsp ground cardamom

⅛ tsp sea salt

METHOD

1 In a large saucepan over medium heat, combine red apples, water, animal fat, cinnamon, allspice, nutmeg, ginger, cloves, cardamom, and sea salt. Cover, and cook, stirring every 5 minutes, for 30 minutes.

2 Uncover, and cook for 5 more minutes to reduce any liquid in the pan. Remove from heat and allow apples to cool for 5 minutes before serving.

3 If not using immediately, allow to cool completely before storing tightly covered in the refrigerator for up to 1 week.

Variation

Chamomile Ginger Applesauce

STAGE 5

INGREDIENTS

1 chamomile tea bag

1 cup hot water

8 medium yellow or green apples, peeled, cored, and quartered

1 tsp lemon zest

¼ cup lemon juice

½ tsp sea salt

1 tbsp peeled and finely grated ginger

¼ cup raw honey

METHOD

1 Steep 1 chamomile tea bag in hot water for 10 minutes, and then discard the tea bag.

2 In a medium stockpot over high heat, combine apples, lemon zest, lemon juice, sea salt, brewed tea, and ginger. Bring to a boil, reduce heat to medium-low, and simmer for 25 minutes or until apples are tender and cooked through.

3 Remove from heat, and mash apples with a potato masher, or process in small batches in a food processor or blender until smooth. When desired texture is achieved, fold in honey.

Apple Pie Stewed Apples

DAIRY FREE

Baked Cinnamon Walnut Apples

Tender, baked apples topped with crunchy nuts and sweet cinnamon—this recipe is a great way to use your seasonal apple crop.

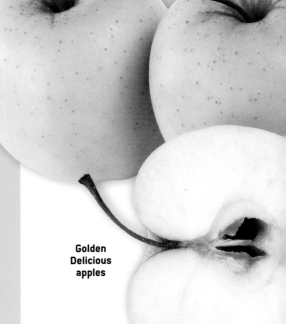

Golden Delicious apples

Prep Time
50 minutes

Cook Time
35 minutes

Makes
4 baked apples

Serving Size
1 baked apple

INGREDIENTS

4 large Rome, Jonagold, Honeycrisp, or Golden Delicious baking apples

4 tsp animal fat (or ghee if dairy is tolerated)

4 tsp raw honey

2 tsp ground cinnamon

$^1/_4$ cup chopped walnuts

$^1/_2$ cup boiling water

METHOD

1 Preheat the oven to 375°F (190°C).

2 Using an apple corer or paring knife, core apples, leaving $^1/_2$ inch (1.25cm) of apple in place at the bottom. Carve the center hole to 1 inch (2.5cm) diameter.

3 In a small bowl, combine animal fat, honey, cinnamon, and walnuts. Evenly divide walnut mixture among 4 apples, spooning into each cored apple center hole.

4 Place apples in an 8×8-inch (20×20cm) baking dish, and pour boiling water in the bottom. Bake on the middle oven rack for 35 minutes or until apples are just tender throughout.

5 Remove from the oven, baste apples with pan juice, and allow to cool 5 minutes before serving.

Variation

Baked Apples with Cinnamon, Walnuts, Raisins, and Yogurt

Add 4 teaspoons unsweetened, unsulfured raisins to the filling and top with 2 tablespoons homemade yogurt when ready to serve.

FULL DIET

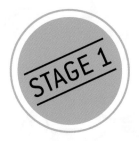

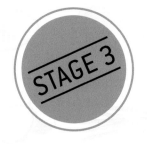

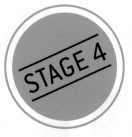

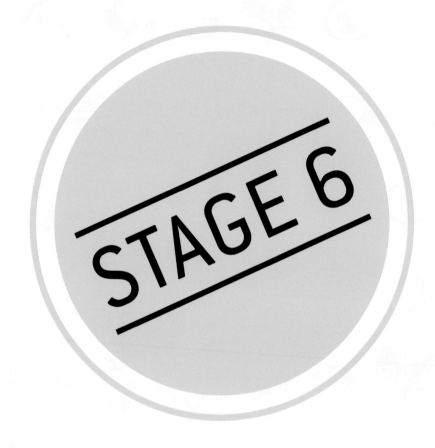

STAGE 6

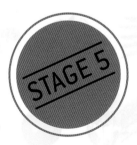

STAGE 5

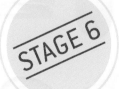

STAGE 6

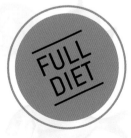

FULL
DIET

Anytime Smoothies

So smooth, creamy, and refreshing, this balanced smoothie is good any time of day. You can vary the berry types and use more of your favorites, or whatever is in season.

Prep Time
5 minutes

Makes
2 smoothies

Serving Size
1 smoothie

INGREDIENTS

1 cup homemade yogurt

$^1/_4$ cup homemade almond milk

$^1/_2$ cup fresh or frozen raspberries, blackberries, blueberries, or strawberries

1 medium banana, sliced ($^1/_2$ cup)

$^1/_4$ cup ripe avocado

$^1/_4$ tsp organic pure vanilla extract

METHOD

1 In a blender, blend homemade yogurt, almond milk, berries, banana, avocado, and vanilla extract for 20 seconds or until smoothie reaches desired consistency.

2 Serve immediately, or refrigerate tightly covered for up to 2 days.

Variations

Cherry Almond Chiller

STAGE 6

Blend 1 cup fresh or frozen cherries, 1 cup homemade almond milk, 3 tablespoons raw soaked and dried whole almonds, 1 tablespoon raw honey, $^1/_2$ teaspoon organic pure almond extract, and 1 tablespoon coconut oil.

PB&J Smoothie

STAGE 6

Blend 1 cup fresh or frozen trimmed and sliced strawberries, 1 cup homemade almond milk, 2 tablespoons all-natural organic peanut butter, 1 tablespoon raw honey, and $^1/_2$ cup sliced banana.

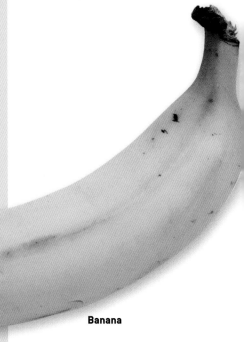

Banana

Roasted Brussels Sprout Apple Salad

Caramelized brussels sprouts, rich and lemony vinaigrette, crunchy almonds, and naturally sweet red apples—this salad is a clean, fresh start to any meal. It's also excellent as a meal itself.

Prep Time	Cook Time	Makes	Serving Size
15 minutes	15 minutes	2 salads	1 salad

INGREDIENTS

3 cups brussels sprouts, stems removed, and quartered

$3/4$ tsp sea salt

2 tsp ghee or animal fat

$1/4$ cup homemade butter, sliced

2 tbsp fresh lemon juice

$1/8$ tsp black pepper

1 medium red apple, cored, quartered, and shaved $1/4$-in (0.5cm) thin

1 thin slice red onion

4 cups baby spinach

3 tbsp slivered almonds

3 tbsp shaved pecorino Romano cheese

METHOD

1 Preheat the oven to 350°F (180°C).

2 In a small bowl, toss together brussels sprouts, $1/4$ teaspoon sea salt, and ghee. Transfer to a large cast-iron skillet or roasting pan, and roast on the top oven rack for 15 minutes or until browned.

3 While sprouts are roasting, heat a light-colored, heavy-bottomed saucepan over medium heat and melt butter, whisking regularly, for 5 minutes. Remove from heat and strain into a small metal bowl. Add lemon juice, $1/4$ teaspoon sea salt, and black pepper, and stir to combine.

4 Remove brussels sprouts from the oven, and cool for 5 minutes.

5 In a medium bowl, combine roasted brussels sprouts, red apple, red onion, baby spinach, almonds, remaining $1/4$ teaspoon sea salt, and pecorino Romano cheese.

6 Drizzle dressing over top, and toss to coat well. Divide salad between two plates, and serve.

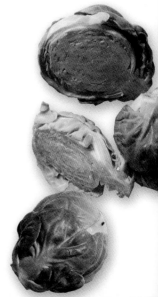

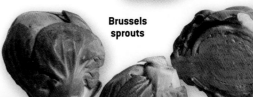

Brussels sprouts

**NUT
FREE**

Scallops Piccata

Sweet caramelized scallops balance nicely with salty capers and a rich and tangy lemon butter sauce. Fresh red tomatoes and chopped Italian flat-leaf parsley lend color to the finished dish.

Prep Time
10 minutes

Cook Time
10 minutes

Makes
16 scallops + sauce

Serving Size
4 scallops + sauce

INGREDIENTS

2 lb (1kg) dry sea scallops

$^1/_4$ tsp sea salt

$^1/_4$ tsp black pepper

2 tbsp ghee

2 cloves garlic

$^1/_4$ cup diced yellow onion

$^1/_2$ cup homemade chicken
 stock

$^1/_4$ cup chopped fresh
 Italian flat-leaf parsley

$^1/_4$ cup fresh lemon juice

2 tbsp caper berries,
 drained

1 cup diced tomato

2 tbsp homemade butter

METHOD

1 Pull side muscles off sea scallops, rinse under cold water, and pat dry. Season both sides of scallops evenly with sea salt and black pepper.

2 Heat a large skillet over medium-high heat, add ghee, and swirl the pan to coat. Add scallops, and cook for 3 minutes per side or until brown and caramelized. Transfer scallops to a plate.

3 Reduce heat to medium, add garlic and yellow onion, and cook for 2 minutes or until onions are just softened.

4 Add chicken stock, and cook for 2 minutes or until reduced by half.

5 Add Italian flat-leaf parsley, lemon juice, caper berries, tomato, and butter, and swirl the pan until butter is incorporated into sauce.

6 Return scallops to the pan, turn to coat, and serve covered with sauce.

> To make this dish low FODMAP, omit the onion and garlic.

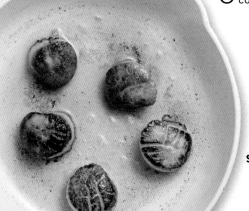

Sea scallops

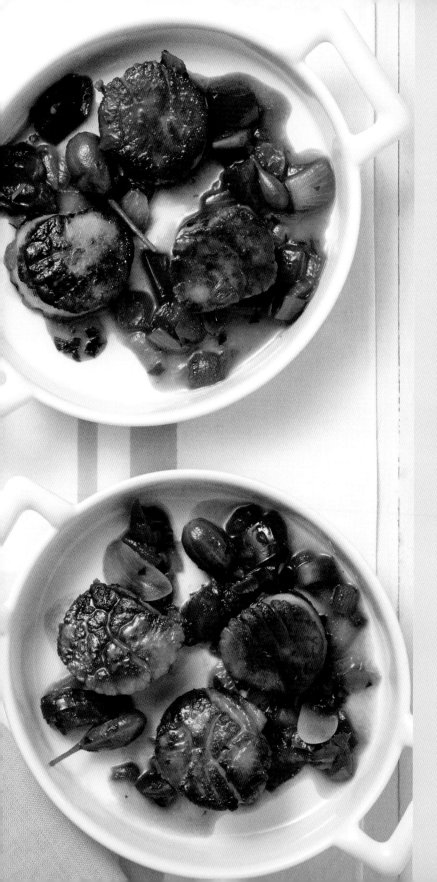

Q&A

What's the difference between wet and dry scallops?

Fishmongers typically sell dry and wet scallops. If they're not labeled as such, be sure to ask. Dry scallops are fresher, have improved flavor, and sear better when cooked. Wet scallops have usually been treated with sodium tripolyphosphate (STP) to help extend their shelf life and maintain moisture. This can make wet scallops difficult to brown when searing, mask their naturally sweet flavor, contribute to a rubbery texture, and release extra fluid during cooking. What's more, STP is a known contributor to inflammation and may impact your gut healing negatively. For best results, buy dry.

DAIRY FREE **NUT FREE** **PALEO DIET**

Olive Raisin Tapenade

Naturally sweet raisins, fruity olives, salty capers, and tangy lemon combine in this amazing spread. Try it on some Three-Seed Crackers for a quick afternoon snack.

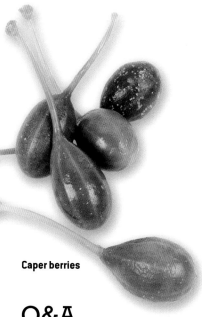

Caper berries

Prep Time
5 minutes

Makes
1 cup

Serving Size
$1/4$ cup

INGREDIENTS

1 cup black olives (no sugar, or other unallowed ingredients, added)

2 tbsp caper berries, drained

$1/4$ cup unsweetened, unsulfured raisins

1 tbsp virgin olive oil

$1/2$ clove garlic

1 tbsp fresh basil leaves

1 tbsp lemon juice

$1/4$ tsp ground black pepper

METHOD

1 In a food processor fitted with a metal chopping blade, process black olives, caper berries, raisins, virgin olive oil, garlic, basil, lemon juice, and black pepper until well blended.

2 Serve immediately or store tightly covered in the refrigerator for up to 1 week.

Q&A

Where else can I use Olive Raisin Tapenade?

Fold this tapenade into your Easy Avocado Omelet at breakfast. Spoon some on salmon or tuna cakes, add a dollop to Greek Lemon Vegetable Soup, add some atop Lamb Burger Sliders, or spread on Oven-Roasted Moroccan Chicken or Lemon Rosemary Salmon. You also can scoop it with raw vegetables, Three-Seed Crackers, and Parmesan Rosemary Tuiles.

NUT FREE

Chicken Thigh Puttanesca

Moist chicken, zesty tomato sauce, bright herbs, and salty Parmesan make this fabulous one-pot meal a favorite.

Prep Time	Cook Time	Makes	Serving Size
15 minutes	15 minutes	8 thighs	2 thighs

INGREDIENTS

- 4 tbsp ghee or animal fat
- 8 bone-in, skin-on chicken thighs (about 3 lb; 1.5kg)
- 1½ tsp sea salt
- 4 cloves garlic, chopped
- 1 cup chopped yellow onion
- ¼ cup caper berries, drained
- 2 cups chopped tomatoes
- 4 oil-packed anchovy fillets, minced
- 4 cups homemade chicken stock
- 1 cup chopped fresh basil leaves
- 2 tbsp chopped fresh oregano leaves
- ¼ cup chopped fresh Italian flat-leaf parsley leaves
- ¼ tsp ground black pepper
- 4 cups tomato purée
- ¼ cup grated Parmesan cheese (optional)

METHOD

1 Heat a Dutch oven with a lid over medium heat. Add 2 tablespoons ghee, and swirl pan to coat bottom.

2 Pat chicken thighs dry, and season with sea salt on both sides. Add chicken, skin side down, and cook for 3 minutes or until lightly browned. Flip over, and cook for 2 minutes or until browned. Transfer chicken to a plate.

3 Add remaining 2 tablespoons ghee, garlic, and yellow onion to the pan, and cook, stirring regularly, for 5 minutes.

4 Add caper berries, tomatoes, anchovies, chicken stock, basil, oregano, parsley, black pepper, and tomato purée, and combine.

5 Return chicken to the pan, and cover with sauce. Bring sauce to a boil, cover, reduce heat to medium-low, and simmer for 30 minutes until it reaches 160°F (70°C). Top with cheese and sauce.

Component

Homemade Fresh Tomato Purée

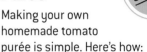

STAGE 1

Making your own homemade tomato purée is simple. Here's how:

1 In a large stockpot over medium-high heat, cook 6 to 8 pounds (2.75–4kg) cored and roughly chopped red ripe plum tomatoes for 10 minutes or until softened.

2 Set a food mill fitted with the largest plate attachment that allows tomatoes but not seeds to pass through over a large bowl, and run tomatoes through.

3 Completely cool tomato purée in an ice bath in the sink before storing tightly covered in nonreactive containers for up to 7 days in the refrigerator or up to 1 year in the freezer.

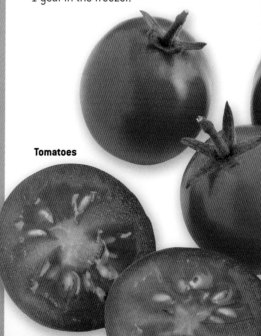

Tomatoes

DAIRY FREE **PALEO DIET**

Dairy-Free Key Lime Mousse

So light, smooth, and tangy with citrus, you'll swear if you close your eyes you can hear the waves crashing onto the sandy island beach. This dessert gets its texture from avocados and bananas rather than dairy ingredients.

Prep Time
20 minutes + 1 hour chill time

Makes
2 cups mousse + 1 cup crust

Serving Size
1/2 cup mousse + 1/4 cup crust

INGREDIENTS

- 1/2 cup walnuts, soaked and dried
- 1/2 cup unsweetened flaked coconut
- 2 medium ripe avocados, peeled and seeded
- 1 medium ripe banana, peeled
- 1 tsp lemon zest (yellow only)
- 2 tbsp fresh lemon juice
- 1 tbsp lime zest (green only)
- 1/4 cup fresh lime juice
- 1 tsp organic pure vanilla extract
- 1/4 cup raw honey
- 1/4 tsp sea salt

METHOD

1 In a food processor fitted with a metal chopping blade, or in a blender, pulse walnuts and coconut until they reach a crumb texture. (Or chop ingredients by hand with a knife.) Transfer mixture to a bowl, and set aside.

2 In the food processor or blender, process avocados, banana, lemon zest, lemon juice, lime zest, lime juice, vanilla extract, honey, and sea salt until smooth. (Or combine by hand with a fork or potato masher.) Refrigerate for at least 1 hour.

3 To serve, place 1/4 cup crust mixture in the bottom of a cup or mug, top with 1/2 cup mousse, and repeat layers to fill. Store unused cups tightly covered in the refrigerator for up to 1 week or in the freezer for up to 1 month.

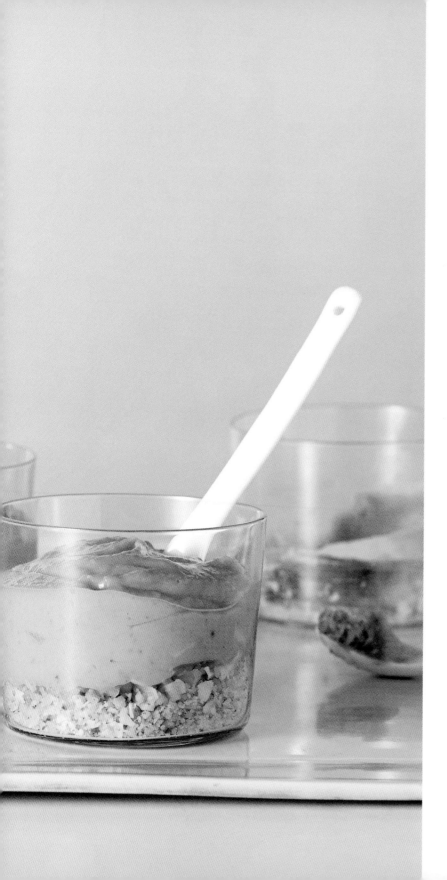

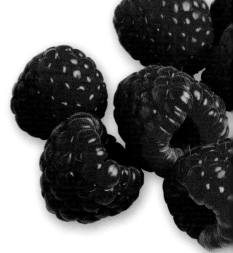

Variation

STAGE 6

Dairy-Free Raspberry Avocado Mousse

Place 2 medium peeled and seeded ripe avocados, 1 frozen peeled banana, $^3/_4$ cup frozen raspberries, 1 tablespoon homemade coconut milk or homemade nut milk, $^1/_4$ cup raw honey, and 1 teaspoon fresh lemon juice in a food processer fitted with a metal blade, and process until smooth. Fill cups or mugs as directed with coconut walnut crumbs, and top with raspberry avocado mousse.

DAIRY FREE **PALEO DIET**

Seasonal Mixed-Berry Crostata

This open-faced baked crostata features a crispy, rustic, free-form crust. Sweet, tangy, seasonal fruit with a hint of cinnamon fills the center.

Prep Time	Cook Time	Makes	Serving Size
15 minutes	50 minutes	8 slices	1 slice

INGREDIENTS

2$^1/_2$ cups fresh seasonal blueberries, raspberries, blackberries, and/or chopped strawberries

1 tsp ground cinnamon

2 tbsp raw honey

1 tsp coconut flour

3 cups almond flour

$^1/_4$ tsp pure baking soda

$^1/_4$ tsp sea salt

$^1/_4$ cup coconut oil, cold and cut into small pieces

1 large egg

METHOD

1 Preheat the oven to 325°F (170°C). Position the oven rack in the center of the oven.

2 In a small bowl, toss berries with $^1/_2$ teaspoon cinnamon, 1 tablespoon raw honey, and coconut flour. Set aside.

3 In a medium bowl, combine almond flour, remaining $^1/_2$ teaspoon cinnamon, baking soda, and sea salt. Add coconut oil, remaining 1 tablespoon honey, and egg, and stir to form a moist dough ball.

4 Place dough in center of a 9-inch (23cm) glass pie plate, and press dough to spread evenly across the bottom of the plate and up the sides. Add berry mixture to center of dough, and carefully fold sides of dough down over berry mixture to cover edges. (It's okay if dough breaks at places while folding.)

5 Bake for about 50 minutes or until crust is uniformly browned and crisp.

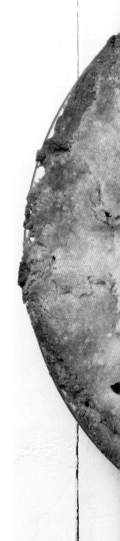

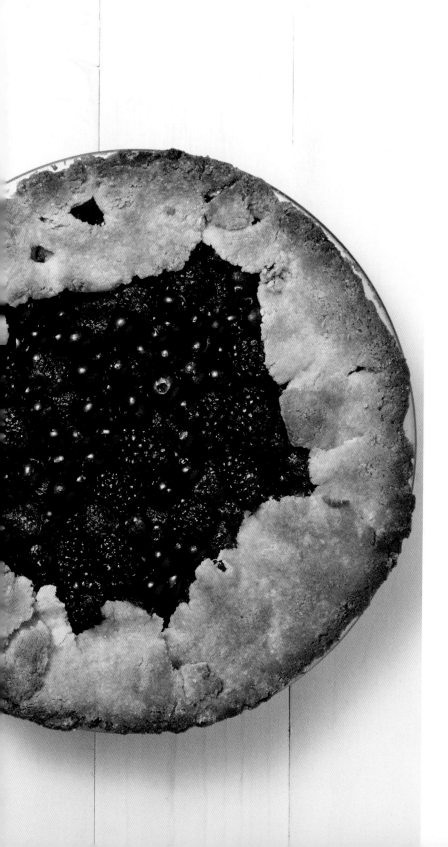

Variation

Cherry Crostata

STAGE 6

Substitute 2$\frac{1}{2}$ cups fresh, stemmed, pitted, and halved cherries for the fresh berries. Continue as directed.

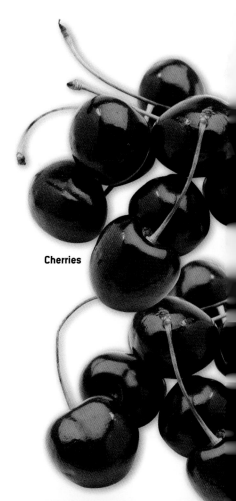

Cherries

DAIRY FREE   **NUT FREE**   **PALEO DIET**

Honey Bombs

These little dessert balls of honey and coconut are subtly sweet and rich in healthy saturated fats. They're fun and easy to make, even for kids.

Prep Time	**Makes**	**Serving Size**
10 minutes	16 pieces	2 pieces

INGREDIENTS

1 1/2 cups coconut butter (also called coconut cream)

1/4 cup unsweetened flaked coconut

1/4 cup coconut flour

1/4 cup raw honey

METHOD

1 In a medium bowl, and using a firm spatula, combine coconut butter, flaked coconut, coconut flour, and honey.

2 Form mixture into 1-tablespoon "bombs," rolling them between your hands into ball shapes.

3 Refrigerate tightly covered for up to 3 months, or freeze for up 6 months.

To make your own coconut flour, pulse 1/4 cup unsweetened flaked coconut in a food processor fitted with a metal chopping blade until it reaches the consistency of flour.

Variation

Chocolate Honey Bombs

STAGE 6

Combine 1/4 cup cocoa powder and 1 teaspoon honey, form into balls, and proceed as described. Be sure you've had 6 months free of digestive symptoms before attempting to reintroduce cocoa because it can cause digestive distress.

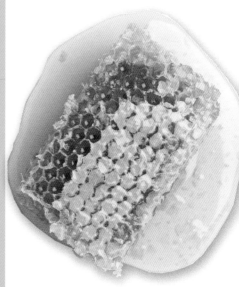

Honey

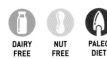

DAIRY FREE **NUT FREE** **PALEO DIET**

Gingered Vanilla Honey Drops

These gut-friendly candies are a satisfying balance between sweet, sour, and spicy. The raw honey delivers antimicrobial benefits, the anti-inflammatory ginger relaxes and soothes the GI tract, and both deliver powerful antioxidants.

Prep Time
5 minutes

Cook Time
15 minutes

Makes
50 drops

Serving Size
1 drop

INGREDIENTS

1 cup raw honey

¼ cup apple cider vinegar

½ tsp ground ginger

¼ tsp organic pure vanilla extract

METHOD

1 In a small saucepan over medium-high heat, whisk together honey, apple cider vinegar, and ginger. Bring to a boil, and cook until liquid reaches 275°F (140C°) on a candy thermometer.

2 Remove from heat, and set aside for 1 minute. Gently stir in vanilla extract.

3 Pour mixture onto a baking sheet lined with parchment paper or into candy molds, and refrigerate for 20 minutes.

4 Cut or break candies into small pieces (if not in molds). Store in a tightly covered container in layers separated by parchment paper.

As long as it's unpasteurized, raw honey has an unlimited shelf life. Raw honey has a low water content and high acidity, which makes a very unfavorable environment for bacteria growth. To maximize quality of raw honey over time, keep it tightly sealed in a dry, room temperature place, like a kitchen cupboard.

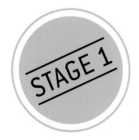

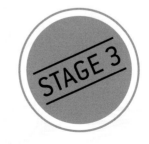
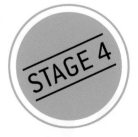

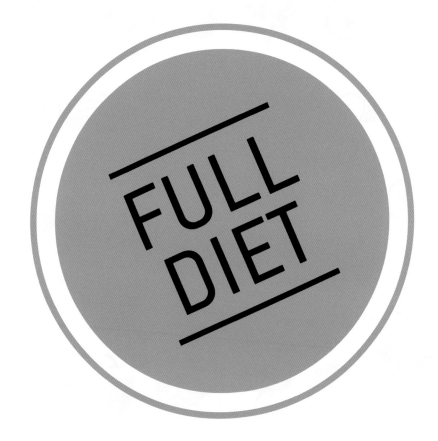

FULL DIET

STAGE 5

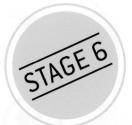

STAGE 6

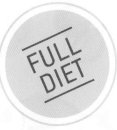

FULL DIET

DAIRY FREE **NUT FREE**

Honey Sage Sausage Patties

Semisweet and savory, these "breakfast burgers" feature a hint of honey and fragrant, warm sage to create pure deliciousness.

Prep Time	**Cook Time**	**Makes**	**Serving Size**
5 minutes	10 minutes	8 patties	1 patty

INGREDIENTS

1 lb (450g) ground pork
2 tsp raw honey
1 tsp pure dry mustard powder
1 tsp pure rubbed sage
1 tsp pure onion powder
$1/4$ tsp pure garlic powder
$1/2$ tsp ground black pepper
$1/2$ tsp sea salt
3 tbsp animal fat (or ghee if dairy is tolerated)

METHOD

1 In a medium bowl, combine pork, honey, dry mustard powder, sage, onion powder, garlic powder, black pepper, and sea salt.

2 Using a $1/4$ cup scoop, form 8 ($1/2$-inch; 1.25cm) patties.

3 In a large skillet over medium heat, heat animal fat, swirling to coat the bottom of the skillet as it melts.

4 Add sausage patties, cover, and cook for 5 minutes.

5 Uncover, carefully turn over patties, recover, and cook for 5 more minutes or until juices run clear.

Variation

Spicy Italian Chicken Sausage Patties

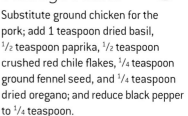

FULL DIET

Substitute ground chicken for the pork; add 1 teaspoon dried basil, $1/2$ teaspoon paprika, $1/2$ teaspoon crushed red chile flakes, $1/4$ teaspoon ground fennel seed, and $1/4$ teaspoon dried oregano; and reduce black pepper to $1/4$ teaspoon.

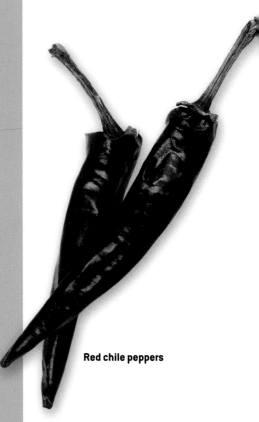

Red chile peppers

NUT
FREE

Sausage, Egg, and Cheese Sandwich

You won't miss fast food when you can make this easy, equally fast sandwich that's gooey, warm, satisfying—and gut friendly.

Prep Time
5 minutes

Cook Time
3 minutes

Makes
1 sandwich

Serving Size
1 sandwich

INGREDIENTS

1 large pastured egg

1/8 tsp sea salt

1 tsp ghee or animal fat

1 slice sharp white cheddar cheese

2 slices grain-free bread, toasted, or 1 Cheddar Chive Biscuit, halved

1 Honey Sage Sausage Patty, cooked

METHOD

1 In a small bowl, whisk egg and sea salt until frothy.

2 In a small skillet over medium heat, heat ghee. Add egg, and cook, continually moving cooked portion to the center of the skillet with a spatula, for 2 or 3 minutes or until no runny egg remains.

3 Place white cheddar cheese slice on 1 piece of bread, top with Honey Sage Sausage Patty, add egg, and top with remaining slice of bread.

Variation

Italian Sausage Egg Sandwich

FULL
DIET

INGREDIENTS

1/4 cup diced yellow onion

1/4 cup diced green bell pepper

1/2 clove garlic, minced

1 tbsp ghee

1 Spicy Italian Chicken Sausage Patty

1 large pastured egg

2 slices shaved Parmesan or Romano cheese

2 slices grain-free bread, toasted

METHOD

1 In a small skillet over medium heat, cook yellow onion, green bell pepper, and garlic in ghee for 5 minutes or until softened.

2 Reheat cooked Spicy Italian Chicken Sausage Patty.

3 Cook egg as directed in step 2.

4 Top sausage patty with Parmesan cheese, egg, bell peppers, onion, and garlic. Place between slices of toasted grain-free bread.

Cheddar Chive Biscuits

You'll love these light and flaky grain-free biscuits. Try them with creamy Sausage Gravy or simply homemade butter.

Prep Time
25 minutes

Cook Time
20 minutes

Makes
8 biscuits

Serving Size
2 biscuits

INGREDIENTS

4 cups almond flour
$^1/_2$ tsp sea salt
$^1/_2$ tsp baking soda
$^1/_3$ cup coconut oil, chilled
$^1/_2$ cup shredded cheddar cheese
$^1/_2$ cup chopped fresh chives
2 large pastured eggs

METHOD

1 Preheat the oven to 400°F (200°C). In a medium bowl, combine almond flour, sea salt, and baking soda.

2 In another medium bowl, whisk together coconut oil, cheddar cheese, chives, and eggs.

3 Slowly add dry ingredients to wet ingredients, and stir until dough forms.

4 Place dough on one side of a piece of parchment paper. Fold the parchment over on top of dough, and roll dough to $^3/_4$ inches (2cm) thick. If dough is sticky, dust with additional flour.

5 Using a biscuit cutter, a 2-inch (5cm) round cookie cutter, or the edge of a drinking glass, cut out biscuits. Place on a baking sheet lined with parchment paper, and bake on the middle oven rack for 20 minutes or until browned. Cool before serving.

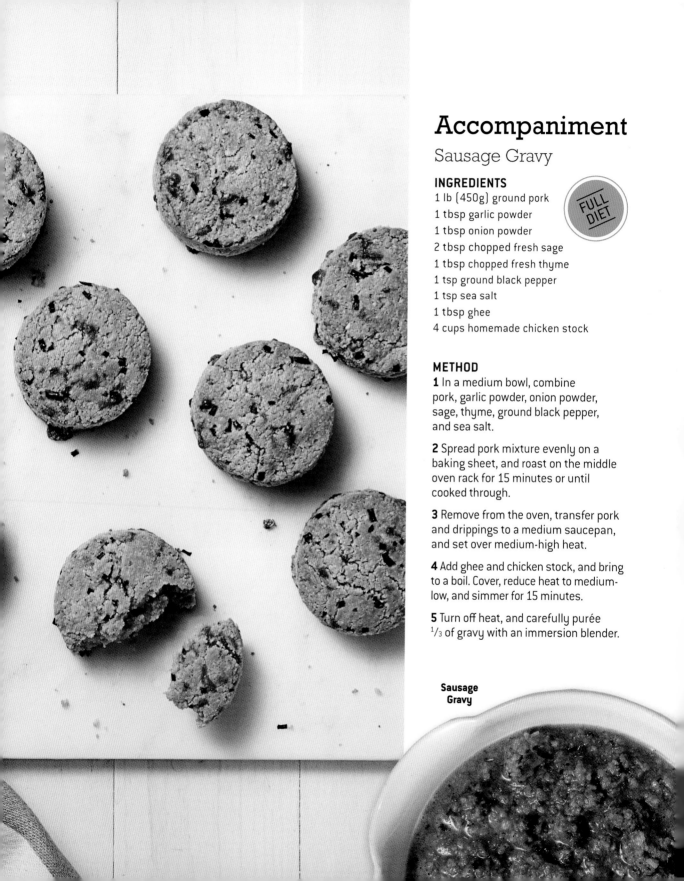

Accompaniment

Sausage Gravy

INGREDIENTS

1 lb (450g) ground pork

1 tbsp garlic powder

1 tbsp onion powder

2 tbsp chopped fresh sage

1 tbsp chopped fresh thyme

1 tsp ground black pepper

1 tsp sea salt

1 tbsp ghee

4 cups homemade chicken stock

FULL DIET

METHOD

1 In a medium bowl, combine pork, garlic powder, onion powder, sage, thyme, ground black pepper, and sea salt.

2 Spread pork mixture evenly on a baking sheet, and roast on the middle oven rack for 15 minutes or until cooked through.

3 Remove from the oven, transfer pork and drippings to a medium saucepan, and set over medium-high heat.

4 Add ghee and chicken stock, and bring to a boil. Cover, reduce heat to medium-low, and simmer for 15 minutes.

5 Turn off heat, and carefully purée 1/3 of gravy with an immersion blender.

Sausage Gravy

DAIRY FREE

PALEO DIET

Grainless Granola

Nuts and seeds are a staple of the healthy gut diet, and this recipe combines their crunchy nuttiness with other gut-supportive ingredients into a delicious, gluten-free, grain-free granola.

Prep Time
5 minutes

Cook Time
40 minutes

Makes
6 cups

Serving Size
1/2 cup

INGREDIENTS

1 cup unsweetened shredded coconut

1/2 cup raw walnuts

1/2 cup raw almonds

1/2 cup raw hazelnuts

1/2 cup raw Brazil nuts

1/2 cup raw cashews

1/2 cup raw pecans

1/2 cup raw shelled sunflower seeds

1/2 cup raw shelled pumpkin seeds

1/3 cup raw honey

1/4 cup coconut oil

2 tsp. pure vanilla extract

1 tsp. ground cinnamon

1/4 tsp sea salt

1/2 cup unsweetened, unsulfured dried apples, peaches, apricots, cherries, raisins, or currants

1/2 cup raw sesame seeds

METHOD

1 Preheat the oven to 300°F (150°C). In a medium bowl, mix coconut, nuts, pumpkin seeds, sunflower seeds, honey, coconut oil, vanilla extract, cinnamon, and sea salt.

2 Transfer to a large baking sheet, spread in an even layer, and bake on the middle oven rack for 20 minutes.

3 Add dried fruit and sesame seeds, stir to combine, and bake for 20 minutes or until toasted.

4 Remove from the oven, and allow to cool completely.

5 Break clusters into smaller pieces as needed, and store in an airtight container in a cool, dry place.

All nuts must be properly soaked and dried, and roughly chopped.

Q&A

How else can I use Grainless Granola?

This versatile granola works great as a breakfast cereal with homemade almond milk, sprinkled on top of homemade yogurt with ground cinnamon and fresh berries for a snack, or on its own by the handful. On the move? Pack some granola to go. It's nonperishable, so it needs no refrigeration when you're out and about!

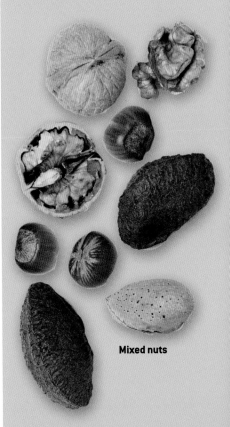
Mixed nuts

DAIRY FREE

NUT FREE

PALEO DIET

Grilled Vegetable Frittata

Grilling adds a smoky flavor to this savory one-pot dish that features a colorful mix of antioxidant-rich vegetables. It's easy to make ahead and great hot or cold.

Prep Time
20 minutes

Cook Time
45 minutes

Makes
8 slices

Serving Size
1 slice

INGREDIENTS

2 cloves garlic, minced

$^1/_2$ tsp sea salt

1 small zucchini, cut into 1-in (2.5cm) slices

1 small yellow summer squash, cut into 1-in (2.5cm) slices

1 medium orange bell pepper, ribs and seeds removed, and cut into 1-in (2.5cm) slices

1 medium red bell pepper, ribs and seeds removed, and quartered

$^1/_2$ cup scallions, white and green parts

1 medium red onion, cut into 1-in (2.5cm) slices

1 tbsp animal fat (or ghee if dairy is tolerated)

12 large eggs

$^1/_4$ cup chopped fresh basil

$^1/_4$ cup chopped fresh Italian flat-leaf parsley

$^1/_2$ cup grated Parmesan cheese

METHOD

1 Preheat the grill to medium. Preheat the oven to 350°F (180°C). Lightly grease a medium ovenproof skillet with animal fat.

2 In a medium bowl, combine garlic, sea salt, and vegetables. Drizzle with animal fat, and toss to coat.

3 Place vegetables on the grill grates, and cook for 3 minutes per side. Transfer to a plate, and then chop and add to skillet. Cool for 15 minutes.

4 In a large bowl, whisk together eggs, basil, parsley, and cheese. Pour over vegetables in the skillet, set over medium-low heat, and cook without stirring for 5 minutes.

5 Transfer the skillet to the oven, and bake for 40 minutes or until set. Turn to broiler setting, and brown for 2 minutes.

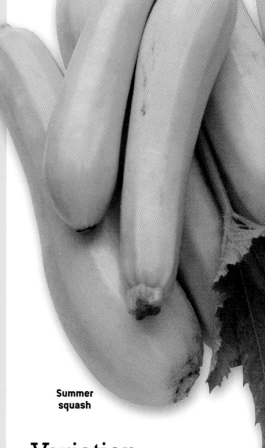

Summer squash

Variation

Roasted Vegetable Frittata

FULL DIET

Preheat the oven to 450°F (230°C). Spread the coated vegetables evenly over a large baking sheet, and roast on the middle oven rack for 10 minutes. Remove from the oven, and allow to cool before roughly chopping and combining with the egg mixture as directed.

DAIRY FREE

NUT FREE

PALEO DIET

Chopped Cobb Salad

A main-dish garden salad made with crispy greens, soft hard-boiled eggs, moist chicken, cool tomatoes, and sharp red onion. This flexible combo salad gives you a little bit of everything.

Prep Time
15 minutes

Makes
2 salads + 1/2 cup dressing

Serving Size
1 salad + 1/4 cup dressing

INGREDIENTS

1/4 cup virgin olive oil

1/4 cup lemon juice

1 tbsp chopped fresh basil, cilantro, or Italian flat-leaf parsley

1/4 tsp sea salt

1/4 tsp black pepper

4 cups chopped romaine lettuce

1 cup cooked and shredded or diced chicken (from stock chicken)

1 medium tomato, diced

1/2 small red onion, diced

1 medium avocado, peeled, pitted, and diced

2 hard-boiled eggs, peeled and sliced

METHOD

1 In a small bowl, whisk together virgin olive oil, lemon juice, basil, sea salt, and black pepper. Set aside.

2 In a large bowl, combine romaine lettuce, chicken, tomato, red onion, and avocado.

3 Add dressing to salad, and toss to coat.

4 Divide dressed salad evenly between 2 bowls, place hard-boiled eggs on the side, and serve.

To hard-boil eggs, place fresh eggs in a large saucepan, cover completely with water, set over high heat, and bring to a boil. Reduce heat to medium-high, and simmer for 9 minutes. Drain and run cold water over eggs until cooled.

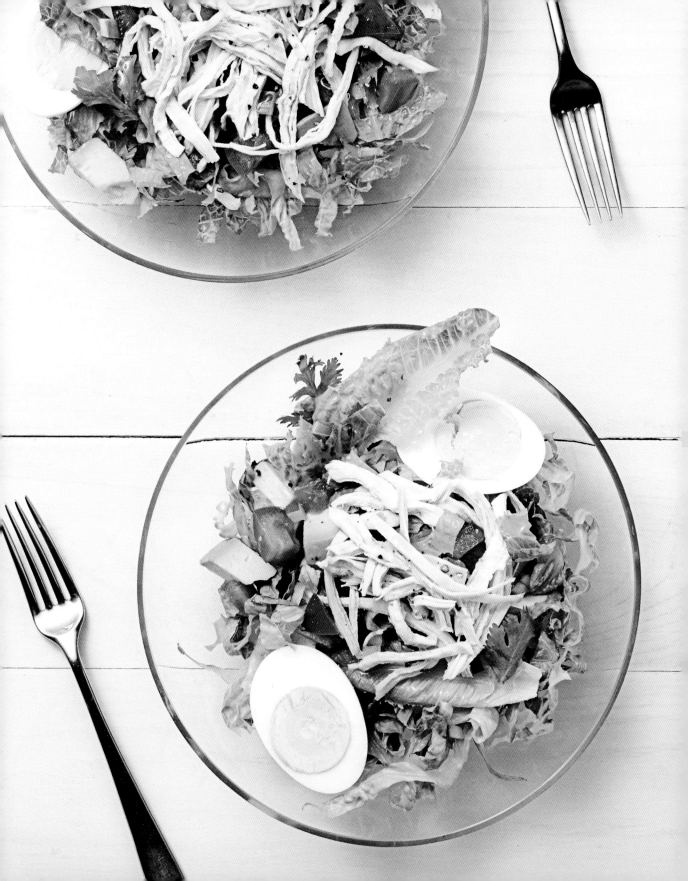

Calming Kale Salad

Kale is a true nutrition powerhouse! Massaging the dressing into the kale "calms" and tenderizes the leaves in this hearty, lemony, and nutty salad. They "relax" even more the longer the salad sits.

Prep Time
15 minutes

Makes
2 salads

Serving Size
1 salad

INGREDIENTS

$^1/_2$ clove garlic, minced

1 cup fresh lemon juice

1 cup virgin olive oil

$^1/_4$ tsp sea salt

$^1/_4$ tsp ground black pepper

6 cups chopped Italian kale, large, tough stems discarded

1 cup chopped grilled or shredded chicken

$^1/_2$ cup peeled, shredded carrots

$^1/_4$ cup chopped raw walnuts

$^1/_4$ cup thinly sliced scallions, green part only

$^1/_4$ cup dried unsweetened, unsulfured currants

2 thin slices red onion

$^1/_4$ cup diced Brie cheese, rind off

METHOD

1 In a small bowl, whisk together garlic, lemon juice, virgin olive oil, sea salt, and black pepper.

2 Place Italian kale in a medium bowl, and drizzle dressing over top. Gently massage dressing into kale leaves for 5 minutes.

3 Add chicken, carrots, walnuts, scallions, currants, red onion, and Brie cheese. Toss to combine, and serve.

4 Refrigerate any unused dressing tightly covered. Shake before serving.

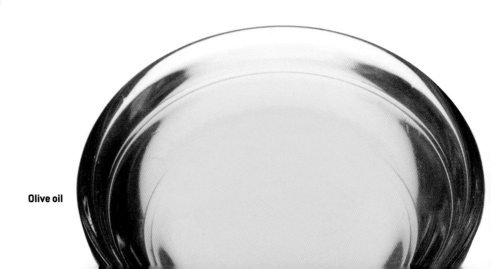

Olive oil

NUT FREE

Grilled Steak Salad

Crispy lettuce, rich and meaty grilled steak and portobellos, tomatoes, and a mildly pungent creamy dressing join to create a salad perfect for a barbecue.

Prep Time	**Cook Time**	**Makes**	**Serving Size**
15 minutes	20 minutes	2 salads	1 salad

INGREDIENTS

- 2 medium portobello mushrooms, stems removed
- 1 tbsp ghee or animal fat
- $1/2$ tsp sea salt
- $1/8$ tsp ground black pepper
- 12 oz (340g) top sirloin steak, 1 to $1^1/2$ in (2.5–3.75cm) thick
- 6 cups chopped romaine lettuce hearts
- 1 medium red ripe tomato, cored and sliced into 4 slices
- $1/2$ avocado, peeled, seeded, and sliced
- 2 thin slices red onion
- $1/2$ cup Horsey Dressing

METHOD

1 Preheat the grill to medium. Brush both sides of portobello mushrooms with ghee, and sprinkle mushroom and steak with salt and pepper.

2 Grill for 7 minutes, rotating 90 degrees midway through cook time. Flip over and cook for 7 minutes on the other side, rotating 90 degrees midway through.

3 Transfer steak and portobellos to separate plates, and let rest for 5 minutes before slicing thinly on the bias.

4 In a medium bowl, toss together romaine lettuce, tomato, avocado, red onion, steak, and portobellos, and toss with Horsey Dressing to coat.

Dressing

Horsey Dressing

FULL DIET

In a food processor fitted with a metal blade, process $1^3/4$ cups homemade yogurt; 4 tablespoons peeled, freshly grated horseradish root; 1 teaspoon lemon juice; $1/4$ cup scallion, green parts only, chopped small; $1/8$ teaspoon black pepper; and $1/4$ teaspoon sea salt until smooth. Refrigerate tightly covered until needed.

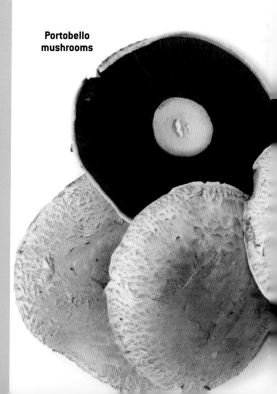

Portobello mushrooms

DAIRY FREE

NUT FREE

PALEO DIET

Seared Scallop Salad with Asian Vegetables

Browned, tender, and mildly sweet scallops are the star in this salad. Crisp, garden-fresh vegetables and a refreshing, citrusy dressing complete this light but satisfying dish that's perfect for a summer dinner.

Prep Time	Cook Time	Makes	Serving Size
20 minutes	5 minutes	4 cups	2 cups

INGREDIENTS

1 cup fresh orange juice

$^2/_3$ cup apple cider vinegar

$^1/_4$ cup tahini paste

$^1/_2$ tsp kosher salt

$^1/_4$ cup fresh cilantro

1 clove garlic

1 cup virgin olive oil

1 small carrot, peeled and grated

1 small red bell pepper, ribs and seeds removed, and sliced thin

3 cups thinly sliced napa cabbage

1 medium scallion, white and green parts, sliced thin on the bias

$^1/_2$ small red onion, sliced thin

8 ($^1/_2$-lb; 225g) dry sea scallops

$^1/_4$ tsp sea salt

1 tbsp animal fat (or ghee if dairy is tolerated)

METHOD

1 In a blender, pulse orange juice, apple cider vinegar, tahini paste, kosher salt, cilantro, and garlic to combine. Turn blender on low speed, and slowly drizzle in virgin olive oil.

2 In a medium bowl, combine carrot, red bell pepper, napa cabbage, scallion, and red onion. Add dressing, and toss to coat.

3 Remove small side muscles from sea scallops, rinse scallops with cold water, and thoroughly pat dry. Sprinkle sea salt over scallops.

4 Heat a medium skillet over medium-high heat, and add animal fat, swirling the skillet to spread. Gently add scallops, and sear scallops for $1^1/_2$ minutes or until a golden crust forms on each side and center is translucent.

5 Divide dressed salad between 2 plates, top each salad with 4 cooked scallops, and serve.

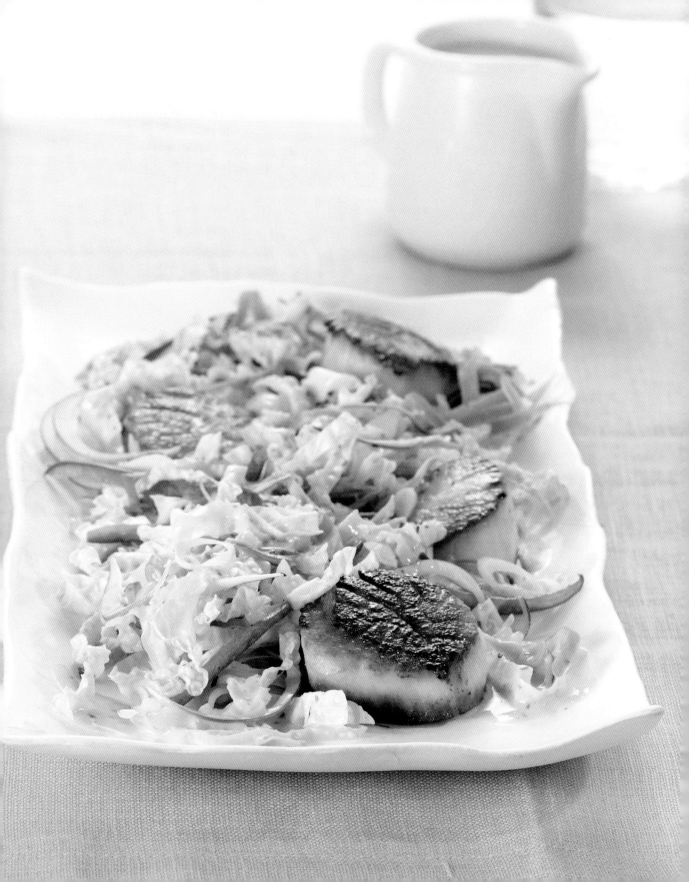

NUT FREE

Wedge Salad with Ranch

Green, leafy lettuce leaves; bright, garden-fresh vegetables; and a light, creamy, herbaceous dressing makes a quick, easy, and delicious salad. Throw in some grilled, poached, or shredded chicken, fish, or beef or some hard-boiled eggs for an added boost of protein.

Prep Time
15 minutes

Makes
4 salads

Serving Size
1 salad

INGREDIENTS

- 1 head Boston, Bibb, or romaine lettuce, soft leaves only
- 1 cup peeled and shredded carrots
- 1 cup halved cherry tomatoes
- 1 cup cucumber, peeled, seeded, halved lengthwise, and sliced
- 2 thin slices red onion
- 1 cup homemade yogurt
- 1 tsp chopped fresh dill
- 1 tsp chopped fresh cilantro
- 1 tsp chopped fresh basil
- 1 tbsp chopped scallion
- $1/2$ clove garlic, minced
- 1 tsp apple cider vinegar
- $1/4$ tsp sea salt
- $1/4$ tsp ground black pepper
- 2 tbsp grated pecorino Romano cheese
- $1/2$ cup virgin olive oil

METHOD

1 Remove tough stems and core from lettuce, and chop into quarters.

2 Place 1 lettuce wedge on each of 4 plates, and top each with carrots, $1/4$ cup cherry tomatoes, $1/4$ cup cucumber, and $1/2$ slice red onion.

3 In a small bowl, combine homemade yogurt, dill, cilantro, basil, scallion, garlic, vinegar, sea salt, ground black pepper, and cheese. Slowly whisk in olive oil until combined. Or place all ingredients in a glass jar with a lid and shake until well combined.

4 Drizzle each salad with $1/4$ cup dressing.

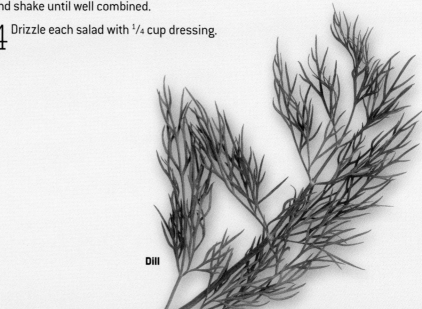

Dill

DAIRY FREE

Spring Tuna Niçoise Salad

In this crispy, crunchy, and colorful nontraditional version of the traditional salad, a tangy and salty vinaigrette ties it all together. You can substitute poached or canned salmon for tuna if you like.

Prep Time
15 minutes

Makes
2 salads

Serving Size
1 salad

INGREDIENTS

$^1/_2$ cup apple cider vinegar

$^1/_2$ cup cool water

$^1/_4$ cup chopped capers

$^1/_4$ cup pitted and chopped Niçoise or Kalamata olives

3 tbsp dry mustard powder

1 tbsp fresh Italian flat-leaf parsley

$^1/_2$ tsp ground black pepper

$^1/_2$ cup virgin olive oil

6 cups chopped red and green leaf lettuce

$^1/_2$ cup thinly sliced red bell pepper

$^1/_2$ cup thinly sliced green scallions

2 thin slices red onion

$^1/_2$ cup cucumber, peeled, seeded, halved, and sliced

$^1/_2$ cup frozen artichoke hearts, thawed and quartered

$^1/_2$ cup halved cherry tomatoes

$^1/_2$ cup thin green beans, cut into 1-in (2.5cm) pieces

2 tsp slivered almonds, soaked and dried

6 oz (170g) tuna packed in oil

METHOD

1 In a blender or a food processor fitted with a metal chopping blade, process apple cider vinegar, cool water, capers, Niçoise olives, dry mustard powder, Italian flat-leaf parsley leaves, and black pepper until smooth.

2 With the processor or blender running on low, drizzle in virgin olive oil until combined.

3 In a medium bowl, combine red and green leaf lettuce, red bell pepper, scallions, red onion, cucumber, artichoke hearts, cherry tomatoes, green beans, almonds, and tuna.

4 Drizzle with 6 tablespoons dressing, toss to coat well. Divide salad evenly among plates.

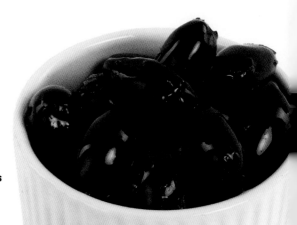

Kalamata olives

DAIRY FREE

PALEO DIET

Salmon Spinach Cobb Salad

This salad offers a ton of variety. Tender baby spinach, rich salmon, crunchy almonds, smooth avocado, and sweet grapes add up to a flavorful and satisfying no-cook meal.

Prep Time
15 minutes

Makes
2 salads

Serving Size
1 salad

INGREDIENTS

4 cups baby spinach

6 oz (170g) canned wild salmon, packed in its juice or oil

$1/4$ cup almonds, soaked, dried, and chopped

$1/2$ medium avocado, peeled, seeded, and sliced

$1/2$ cup halved red seedless grapes

$1/2$ cup thinly sliced red onion

2 Roma tomatoes, quartered

$1/2$ cup cucumber, halved and sliced thin

2 large pastured hard-boiled eggs, peeled and sliced

$1/2$ cup Honey Mustard Vinaigrette

METHOD

1 Divide baby spinach between 2 medium bowls.

2 Evenly divide salmon, almonds, avocado, red grapes, red onion, Roma tomatoes, cucumber, eggs, and Honey Mustard Vinaigrette between bowls, and serve.

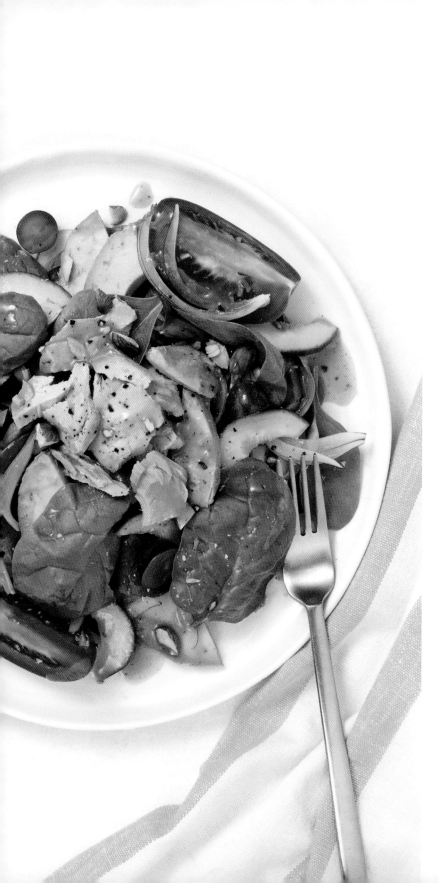

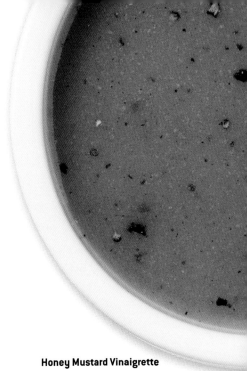

Honey Mustard Vinaigrette

Dressing

Honey Mustard Vinaigrette

For 2 cups vinaigrette, place $^1/_2$ cup raw honey, $^1/_2$ cup apple cider vinegar, $^1/_2$ cup virgin olive oil, $^1/_4$ cup dry mustard powder, 1 tablespoon turmeric powder, 1 tablespoon garlic powder, 2 teaspoons onion powder, 1 teaspoon ground black pepper, and 1 teaspoon sea salt in a glass jar. Seal with the lid, and shake to combine.

STAGE 6

DAIRY FREE **PALEO DIET**

Chunky Chicken Salad

Nothing beats a simple and refreshing chicken salad. Pair with two slices of Everyday Grain-Free Bread for a satisfying sandwich.

Prep Time
10 minutes

Makes
4 cups

Serving Size
1/2 cup

INGREDIENTS

1 large pastured egg

1 tbsp fresh lemon juice

1/4 tsp dry mustard powder

1/4 tsp sea salt

1 cup virgin olive oil

3 cups poached, grilled, or shredded chicken, cooled and diced

1/2 cup quartered red grapes

1/4 cup walnuts, soaked and dried, and chopped

1/4 cup chopped scallions

1/4 cup diced celery

2 tbsp fresh Italian flat-leaf parsley leaves, chopped

1 tbsp fresh lemon juice

1 tsp sea salt

1/4 tsp black pepper

METHOD

1 *For Mayo-Nays:* In a blender or a food processor fitted with a metal blade, combine egg, lemon juice, mustard powder, and sea salt until smooth. On low speed, slowly drizzle in olive oil until emulsified.

2 In a medium bowl, combine chicken, red grapes, walnuts, scallions, celery, Italian flat-leaf parsley, Mayo-Nays, lemon juice, sea salt, and black pepper.

3 Serve on bread, and refrigerate any leftovers tightly covered for up to 1 week.

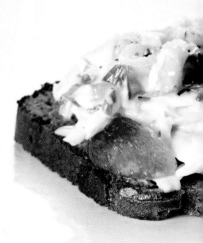

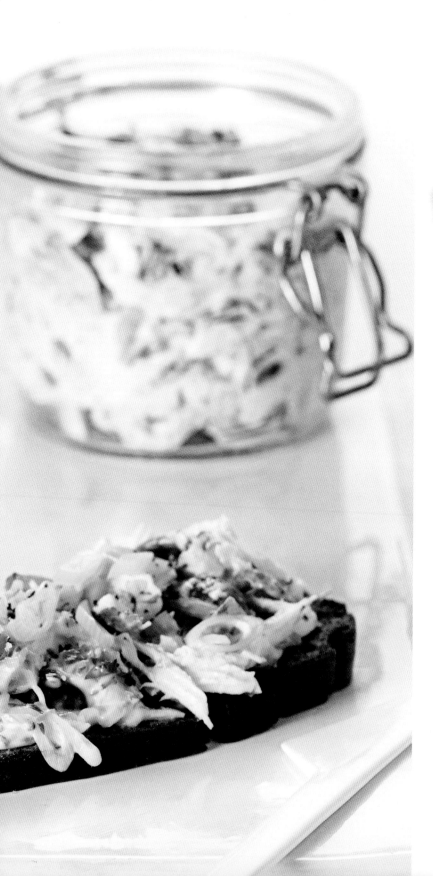

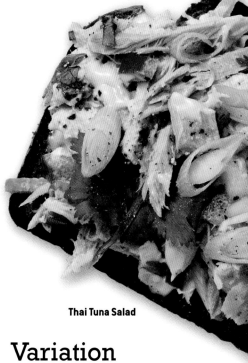

Thai Tuna Salad

Variation

Thai Tuna Salad

STAGE 6

INGREDIENTS

3 cups tuna packed in
 water or its own juices

$1/4$ cup diced red bell pepper

$1/4$ cup chopped scallions

$1/4$ cup peeled, seeded, and
 diced cucumber

$1/4$ cup peeled and shredded
 carrots

2 tbsp chopped fresh cilantro
 leaves

1 tbsp chopped fresh basil
 leaves

1 tbsp fresh lemon juice

$3/4$ cup Mayo-Nays

1 tsp sesame oil

1 tsp sea salt

$1/4$ tsp black pepper

METHOD

In a medium bowl, mix tuna, red bell
pepper, scallions, cucumber, carrots,
cilantro, basil, lemon juice, Mayo-
Nays, sesame oil, sea salt, and black
pepper. Serve on bread. Refrigerate
any leftovers.

NUT
FREE

Chicken Cheddar Sandwiches

Slightly smoky grilled chicken, sharp melted cheddar, toasted bread, and creamy coleslaw make this sandwich a solid addition to your culinary repertoire.

Prep Time	**Cook Time**	**Makes**	**Serving Size**
10 minutes	12 minutes	2 sandwiches	1 sandwich

INGREDIENTS

$1/4$ tsp sea salt

2 (6-oz; 170g) organic boneless, skinless chicken breasts

4 slices grain-free bread

2 slices sharp white cheddar cheese

$2/3$ cup Creamy Coleslaw

METHOD

1 Preheat the grill to medium. Sprinkle sea salt evenly over all sides of chicken.

2 Grill chicken for 6 minutes, rotating 90 degrees halfway through the cook time. Flip over chicken, and cook for 6 minutes, rotating 90 degrees halfway through the cook time, or until internal temperature reaches 160°F (70°C) and juices run clear.

3 Place grain-free bread on the grill, and lightly toast for 3 minutes.

4 Transfer toast to separate plates, and top each of 2 pieces with 1 slice white cheddar cheese, followed by 1 chicken breast, $1/3$ cup Creamy Coleslaw, and remaining piece of toast.

Component

Creamy Coleslaw

FULL DIET

INGREDIENTS

$1/2$ cup homemade mayonnaise or aioli

2 tsp apple cider vinegar

2 tsp raw honey

$1/4$ tsp sea salt

3 cups cored and shredded green cabbage

$1/2$ cup cored and shredded red cabbage

$1/2$ cup peeled and shredded carrots

METHOD

1 In a small bowl, whisk together mayonnaise or aioli, vinegar, honey, and sea salt. In a medium bowl, combine green cabbage, red cabbage, and carrots.

2 Pour dressing over vegetables, and toss well. Refrigerate unused coleslaw tightly covered. (Makes 4 cups.)

Apple cider vinegar

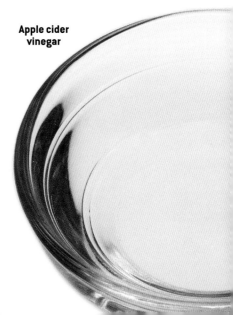

Turkey Reubens

The perfect balance of melted Swiss cheese, tangy sauerkraut, toasty bread, creamy dressing, and thinly sliced turkey, this fantastic deli sandwich hits the spot.

Prep Time	**Cook Time**	**Makes**	**Serving Size**
8 minutes	5 minutes	2 sandwiches	1 sandwich

INGREDIENTS

4 slices grain-free bread

1 tbsp ghee

6 oz (170g) cooked and thinly sliced or shaved turkey or chicken

2/3 cup homemade sauerkraut, drained

2 slices Swiss cheese

4 tbsp Russian Dressing

METHOD

1 Brush one side of each slice of grain-free bread with ghee to coat.

2 Heat a medium skillet over low heat. Place bread slices, ghee side down, in the skillet. Top 2 slices of bread with 3 ounces (85g) turkey each followed by 1/3 cup sauerkraut.

3 Place 1 Swiss cheese slice on each empty bread slice.

4 Cover the skillet with a lid, and cook for 3 to 5 minutes or until turkey and sauerkraut are warmed and cheese is melted.

5 Uncover, and spread 2 tablespoons Russian Dressing on each bread slice with melted cheese.

6 Flip each bread slice with cheese and dressing over onto a slice with turkey and sauerkraut. Transfer sandwiches to a plate, and cut in half if desired.

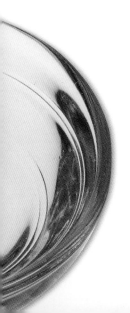

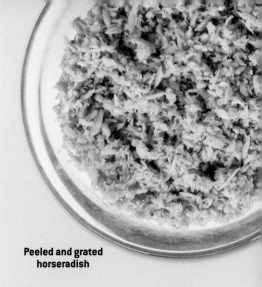

Peeled and grated horseradish

Dressing

Russian Dressing

FULL DIET

INGREDIENTS

1 tbsp finely chopped yellow onion

1 cup homemade Mayo-Nays or aioli

1/4 cup pure tomato paste

1 tbsp raw honey

1 tbsp peeled and finely grated horseradish root

1 tsp apple cider vinegar

1/4 tsp sweet paprika

1/4 tsp sea salt

METHOD

In a small bowl, whisk together yellow onion, Mayo-Nays, tomato paste, raw honey, horseradish root, apple cider vinegar, sweet paprika, and sea salt. (Makes 1 cup.)

DAIRY FREE

Lamb Burger Sliders

Satisfy your appetite with a few of these warm and juicy petite burgers topped with creamy aioli for an added luscious, good-for-your-gut meal.

Prep Time
20 minutes

Cook Time
10 minutes

Makes
8 burgers

Serving Size
2 burgers

INGREDIENTS

1 lb (450g) ground lamb

1 tsp sea salt

16 slices gluten-free bread, lightly toasted

16 thin slices cucumber

8 thin slices tomato

4 thin slices red onion

1 cup Cumin Mint Aioli

METHOD

1 Form lamb into 8 (2-ounce; 55g) patties, and season both sides with sea salt.

2 Heat a large skillet over medium-high heat, add patties, and cook for 3 minutes per side or until patties are cooked through and no pink remains.

3 Set 1 patty on 1 piece of bread. Top with 2 slices cucumber, 1 slice tomato, $^{1}/_{2}$ slice red onion, and 2 tablespoons Cumin Mint Aioli. Add second piece of bread, and serve.

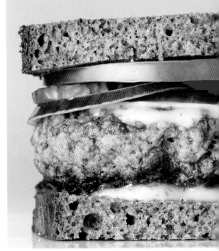

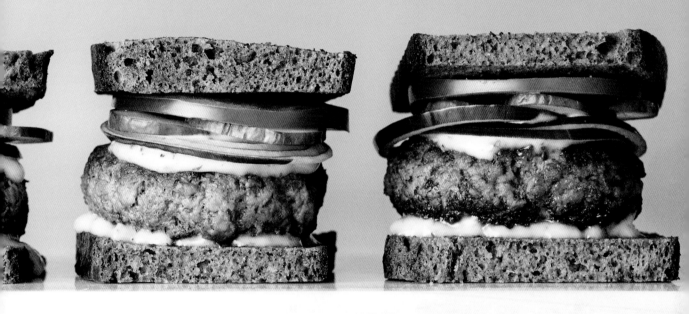

Sauce

Cumin
Mint Aioli

FULL
DIET

INGREDIENTS
1 large pastured egg
1 tbsp fresh lemon juice
$^1/_4$ tsp dry mustard powder
$^1/_4$ tsp sea salt
$^1/_4$ tsp ground black pepper
$^1/_4$ cup fresh mint leaves
1 tsp ground cumin
1 cup virgin olive oil

METHOD
1 In a blender or a food processor
fitted with a metal blade, process
egg, lemon juice, mustard powder,
sea salt, ground black pepper, mint
leaves, and cumin until smooth.

2 With the blender on low speed,
slowly drizzle in olive oil until
emulsified. Refrigerate tightly
covered for up to 1 week.

**Cumin Mint
Aioli**

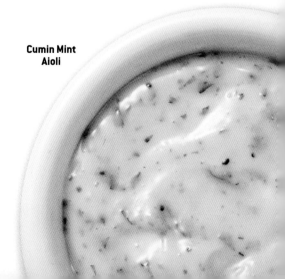

NUT FREE

Margherita Pizza

You don't always get pizza or even cheese on the healthy gut diet. But this GAPS-friendly gluten-free treat delivers a gooey, cheesy goodness you'll love.

Prep Time
10 minutes

Cook Time
25 minutes

Makes
1 (6-slice) pizza

Serving Size
1 slice

INGREDIENTS

1 cup homemade coconut flour

$1/2$ cup coconut oil

6 large pastured eggs

1 tsp sea salt

1 tsp pure garlic powder

1 tsp pure onion powder

$1/2$ cup tomato purée

1 medium tomato, sliced

$3/4$ cup shredded Monterey Jack cheese

1 tbsp grated pecorino Romano cheese

$1/4$ cup chopped fresh basil leaves

METHOD

1 Preheat the oven to 350°F (180°C). Line a baking sheet with parchment paper.

2 In a medium bowl, with a mixer on medium speed, combine coconut flour, coconut oil, eggs, $3/4$ teaspoon sea salt, garlic powder, and onion powder for 4 minutes or until soft and smooth.

3 Transfer dough to the baking sheet, and press to a 9-inch (23cm) diameter, $1/2$-inch (1.25cm) thick circle. Bake for 10 minutes.

4 Remove baking sheet from the oven, place a second piece of parchment paper on top of crust, and carefully flip over crust so new paper is now on the bottom. Bake 8 more minutes.

5 Spread tomato purée evenly over top of cooked crust. Top with tomatoes, salt, and cheese.

6 Bake 5 more minutes and top with basil.

Variations

Philly Cheesesteak Pizza

FULL DIET

Top the shell evenly with $1/2$ cup tomato purée, $1/2$ cup cooked and shredded beef, $1/4$ cup sautéed sliced yellow onion, $1/4$ cup sliced brown button mushrooms, and $1/4$ cup seeded and sliced green bell peppers. Top with $3/4$ cup shredded white cheddar cheese, and bake as directed.

Chicken Parmesan Pizza

FULL DIET

Top the shell evenly with $1/2$ cup tomato purée, $1/2$ cooked and chopped chicken, and $1/2$ cup shaved Parmesan cheese, and bake as directed. Top with 2 tablespoons chopped fresh basil leaves.

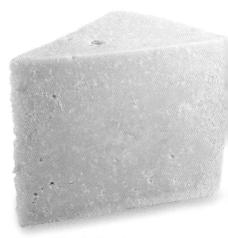

White cheddar cheese

DAIRY FREE

Tuna Cakes with Rémoulade

Golden, lemony, and moist, these mild tuna cakes will tame even the pickiest of fish eaters. Double the tuna cake size and you can use the cakes in a sandwich.

Prep Time 20 minutes

Cook Time 15 minutes

Makes 12 cakes + 1 cup dressing

Serving Size 3 cakes + ¹/₄ cup dressing

INGREDIENTS

³/₄ cup homemade aioli or Mayo-Nays

1 tbsp grain mustard

1 tbsp capers, drained

1 tbsp chopped red onion

1 tbsp chopped scallion, green part only

1 tsp apple cider vinegar

³/₄ tsp sea salt

¹/₄ tsp ground black pepper

18 oz (510g) canned or jarred tuna

3 large pastured eggs

¹/₂ cup diced yellow onion

2 tbsp fresh lemon juice

3 tbsp chopped fresh Italian flat-leaf parsley leaves

1 tsp minced garlic

¹/₂ cup coconut oil (or ghee if dairy is tolerated)

METHOD

1 *For Grain Mustard Rémoulade:* In a food processor, chop aioli, grain mustard, capers, red onion, scallion, apple cider vinegar, ¹/₄ teaspoon sea salt, and black pepper until just smooth.

2 In a medium bowl, combine tuna, eggs, yellow onion, lemon juice, Italian flat-leaf parsley, garlic, and remaining ¹/₂ teaspoon sea salt. Form into 12 patties ³/₄ inch (2cm) thick.

3 In a large skillet over medium heat, heat ¹/₄ cup coconut oil. Add 6 tuna cakes to the skillet, and cook for 3 minutes on each side or until just browned. Transfer cooked cakes to a plate, and repeat with remaining ¹/₄ cup coconut oil and remaining 6 tuna cakes.

4 Serve cooked cakes with Grain Mustard Rémoulade.

Side Dish

Warm Portobello, Red Bell Pepper, and Basil Salad

STAGE 3

INGREDIENTS

¹/₄ cup ghee

3 large portobello mushrooms, stems off, halved, and sliced thin

1 clove garlic, minced

¹/₂ tsp sea salt

¹/₄ tsp ground black pepper

1 large red bell pepper, ribs and seeds removed, halved, and sliced thin

¹/₂ cup chopped fresh basil

METHOD

1 In a large skillet over medium-high heat, heat ghee. Add portobello mushrooms, and cook, stirring regularly, for 3 minutes.

2 Add garlic, sea salt, black pepper, and red bell pepper, and cook for 3 minutes or until bell pepper is softened.

3 Turn off heat, fold in basil, and serve. (Makes 4 cups.)

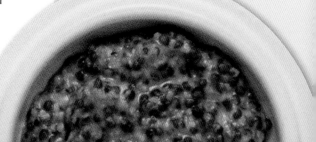

Grain mustard

**DAIRY
FREE**

**NUT
FREE**

**PALEO
DIET**

Oven-Roasted Moroccan Chicken

Citrusy lemon and cilantro blend well with sweet-smelling spices to create a chermoula, a Moroccan marinade, that makes this roasted chicken dish succulent and aromatic.

Prep Time
20 minutes + 4 hours marinate time

Cook Time
60 minutes

Makes
4 leg quarters

Serving Size
1 leg quarter

INGREDIENTS

1 small yellow onion, diced
  (1/2 cup)
6 cloves garlic, chopped
1 cup tomato purée
1/4 cup lemon juice
2 tbsp animal fat (or ghee
  if dairy is tolerated)
1/2 cup chopped fresh
  cilantro
1 tbsp paprika
1 tsp sea salt
1 tsp grated ginger
1 tsp black pepper
1/2 tsp ground cumin
1/2 tsp ground turmeric
4 skin-on, bone-in chicken
  leg quarters (about
  2 lb; 1kg)

METHOD

1 In a large bowl, whisk together yellow onion, garlic, tomato purée, lemon juice, animal fat, cilantro, paprika, sea salt, ginger, black pepper, cumin, and turmeric.

2 Add chicken leg quarters, and coat with spice mix marinade. Cover the bowl tightly with lid, aluminum foil, or plastic wrap, and refrigerate for 4 hours or overnight. Because the raw chicken was sitting in the marinade, do not reuse it at the table as a sauce. Doing so increases the risk of food-borne illness. Instead, double the marinade recipe, set aside half of it, and use it as a condiment.

3 Preheat the oven to 350°F (180°C). Remove chicken leg quarters from marinade, and place skin side up and spaced equally apart in a 9×13-inch (23×33cm) glass baking dish.

4 Bake on the middle oven rack for 60 minutes or until chicken is cooked through or it reaches an internal temperature of 165°F (75°C) and juice runs clear.

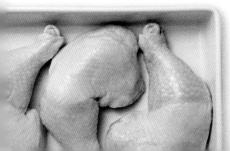

**Arrange the chicken leg
quarters in a baking
dish for even cooking**

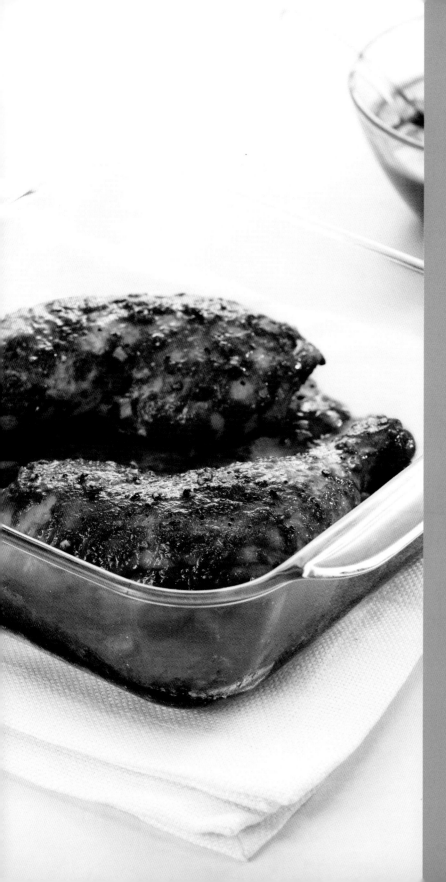

Side Dish

Moroccan Cauliflower "Couscous"

FULL DIET

INGREDIENTS

4 tbsp ghee or animal fat

$\frac{1}{4}$ cup thinly sliced scallions, green and white parts

3 cloves garlic, minced

$\frac{1}{4}$ cup unsweetened, unsulfured raisins

$\frac{1}{4}$ cup slivered almonds

3 tbsp fresh orange juice

2 tsp orange zest

1 cup homemade chicken stock

1 medium head cauliflower, stemmed, cored, grated (4 cups)

1 tbsp Ras el Hanout

1 tsp sea salt

1 tsp apple cider vinegar

METHOD

1 In a medium saucepan over medium-high heat, combine ghee, scallions, garlic, raisins, almonds, orange juice, orange zest, chicken stock, grated cauliflower, Ras el Hanout, sea salt, and apple cider vinegar.

2 Bring to a boil, cover, reduce heat to medium-low, and simmer for 2 minutes. Uncover, and cook, stirring occasionally, for 1 or 2 more minutes or until liquid is cooked away. (Makes 4$\frac{1}{2}$ cups.)

DAIRY FREE **NUT FREE** **PALEO DIET**

Slammin' Hot Slaw

If you like spice, you'll love this slaw. It's crunchy, citrusy, smoky—and hot! It goes great on grilled fish.

Prep Time
15 minutes

Makes
8 cups

Serving Size
3/4 cup

INGREDIENTS

- 3/4 cup homemade aioli or mayonnaise
- 2 tbsp raw honey
- 1 tbsp pure chipotle powder
- 2 tbsp apple cider vinegar
- 2 tbsp fresh lime juice
- 1/2 tsp sea salt
- 1/4 tsp ground black pepper
- 5 cups shredded green cabbage
- 1 cup shredded purple cabbage
- 1 small yellow bell pepper, ribs and seeds removed, halved, and sliced thin
- 1 small red bell pepper, ribs and seeds removed, halved, and sliced thin
- 1 cup thinly sliced scallions
- 1/2 cup peeled and shredded carrots
- 1/2 cup chopped fresh cilantro leaves
- 1 clove garlic, minced
- 1 cup orange segments
- 1 cup halved cherry tomatoes
- 2 jalapeños, stem off and sliced thin

METHOD

1 In a small bowl, whisk together aioli, honey, chipotle powder, apple cider vinegar, lime juice, sea salt, and black pepper.

2 In a large bowl, combine green cabbage, purple cabbage, yellow bell pepper, red bell pepper, scallions, carrots, cilantro, garlic, orange segments, cherry tomatoes, and jalapeños.

3 Add dressing to cabbage mixture, and toss to combine.

4 Refrigerate, tightly covered, for 1 hour before serving.

Q&A

How do I adjust the heat?

To increase the hotness factor of this recipe, substitute habanero or scotch bonnet peppers for the jalapeños. To tone things down a bit, eliminate the seeds and ribs from the jalapeños, substitute Anaheim or Spanish pimentos, cut back on the chipotle powder amount, or substitute smoked paprika for the chipotle.

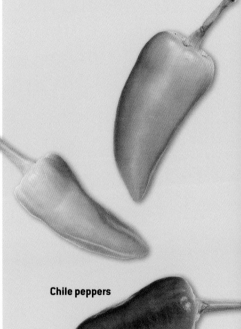

Chile peppers

NUT
FREE

Shrimp and Cauliflower Grits

This low-country star boasts soft, cheesy, buttery cauliflower grits under rich shrimp and a savory tomato sauce. It's a homey comfort dish great for any meal.

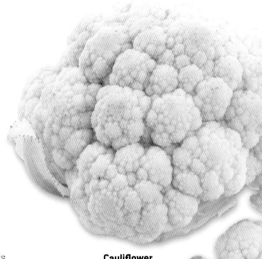

Cauliflower

Prep Time
10 minutes

Cook Time
20 minutes

Makes
16 shrimp + 4 cups grits

Serving Size
4 shrimp + 1 cup grits

INGREDIENTS

1 large head cauliflower, cut into 1-in (2.5cm) florets

4 tbsp ghee or animal fat

2 cloves garlic, minced

$1/4$ cup yellow onion, diced

1 to $1^1/4$ lb (450–565g) fresh shrimp (16 to 20 count; about 16), peeled, deveined, and tail off

1 tbsp lemon juice

$1/2$ cup tomato purée

$3/4$ tsp sea salt

$1/2$ tsp ground black pepper

1 tbsp chopped fresh oregano leaves

$3/4$ cup homemade chicken stock

2 tbsp chopped fresh Italian flat-leaf parsley leaves

$1/3$ cup virgin olive oil

2 tbsp chopped scallion, green parts

$1/2$ cup grated pecorino Romano cheese

METHOD

1 In a large saucepan over medium-high heat, bring 1 cup water to a boil. Reduce heat to medium, place a steamer insert in the pan, and steam cauliflower florets for 20 minutes.

2 In a large skillet over medium heat, heat 2 tablespoons ghee. Add 1 clove garlic, yellow onion, and shrimp, and cook, stirring regularly, for 3 minutes.

3 Add lemon juice, tomato purée, $1/4$ teaspoon sea salt, $1/4$ teaspoon black pepper, oregano, and $1/2$ cup chicken stock. Cook, stirring regularly, for 5 minutes.

4 Remove from heat, fold in Italian flat-leaf parsley, cover, and set aside.

5 Drain cauliflower in a colander and transfer to a food processor fitted with a metal chopping blade. Add remaining $1/4$ cup chicken stock, remaining 1 clove garlic, remaining 2 tablespoons ghee, remaining $1/2$ teaspoon sea salt, remaining $1/4$ teaspoon black pepper, and virgin olive oil, and process until smooth.

6 Transfer cauliflower grits to a bowl, fold in scallions and pecorino Romano cheese, and serve shrimp on top of or alongside grits.

DAIRY FREE

NUT FREE

PALEO DIET

Kimchi

This crispy and flavorful condiment offers hints of salty, sweet, spicy, and sour in each gut-nourishing bite. It's sure to win over the greatest ferment skeptic, and it'll soon become one of your staple recipes.

Prep Time	**Cook Time**	**Makes**	**Serving Size**
20 minutes	7 days	2 (1-quart; 1-liter) jars	¼ cup

INGREDIENTS

- 2 small heads napa cabbage, shredded
- 2 medium red bell peppers, ribs and seeds removed, and sliced thin
- 2 cups red or daikon radishes, sliced thin
- 4 medium carrots, grated
- ¼ cup peeled and grated ginger
- 6 cloves garlic, sliced thin
- 4 scallions, green and white parts, sliced thin
- 2 tsp Korean fish sauce, GAPS legal, no-sugar-added, rating of N30 or higher
- 3 tbsp sea salt
- Spring or filtered water

METHOD

1 In a large bowl, combine napa cabbage, red bell peppers, red radishes, carrots, ginger, garlic, scallions, and Korean fish sauce. Add sea salt, and massage salt into vegetables until vegetables get softer and liquid brine stops forming in bowl.

2 Using a wooden spoon, evenly pack vegetables and liquid brine into 1-quart (1-liter) glass jars, packing down vegetables so they're completely submerged, and leaving at least 1 inch (2.5cm) space at the top of the jar. Add spring water, if necessary, to cover.

3 Cover the jars with lids, and set aside at room temperature out of direct sunlight for 7 days.

4 Once daily, loosen the lids to allow gases to escape. Press down on vegetables as needed to ensure they remain submerged in brine. Retighten the lids. Refrigerate for up to 6 months.

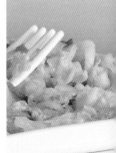

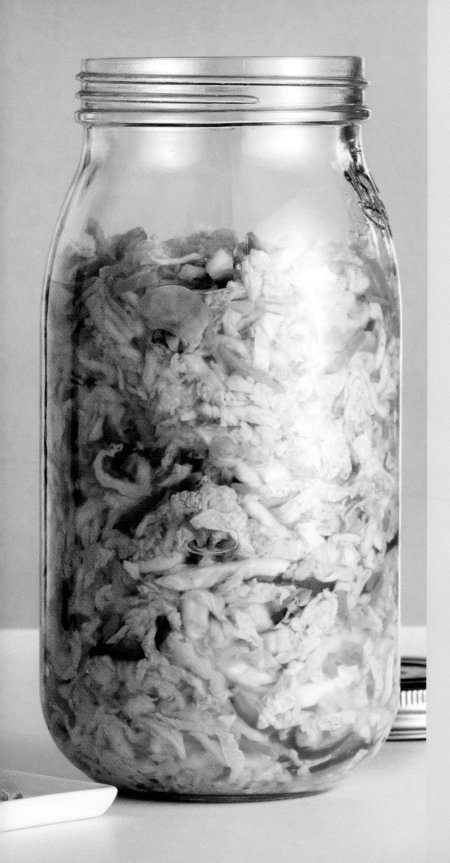

Variation

Kowabunga
Kimchi

Add 1 teaspoon Korean
chile powder or flakes or
1 (or more) fresh chopped red Thai or
red jalapeño chiles to the vegetable mix.

FULL
DIET

DAIRY FREE

NUT FREE

PALEO DIET

Cauliflower Hummus

This soft, toasted, slightly lemony Mediterranean purée makes a great sandwich spread or dip. This version substitutes cauliflower for the traditional chickpeas. Who says white foods can't be great for you?

Prep Time	Cook Time	Makes	Serving Size
15 minutes	20 minutes	4 cups	½ cup

INGREDIENTS

1 large head cauliflower, trimmed of hard stems, leaves, and core, and cut into medium florets

½ cup tahini paste

¼ cup virgin olive oil

1 clove garlic

1 tsp pure ground cumin

2 tbsp lemon juice

1 tsp sea salt

¼ tsp black pepper

METHOD

1 In a large saucepan over medium-high heat, bring 1 cup water to a boil.

2 Reduce heat to medium, and place a steamer insert in the pan. Add cauliflower, cover, and cook for 20 minutes or until cauliflower is soft and fork-tender. Drain cauliflower into a colander, and cool completely.

3 In a food processor fitted with a metal chopping blade, purée cooled cauliflower, tahini paste, virgin olive oil, garlic, cumin, lemon juice, sea salt, and black pepper until smooth.

4 Keep tightly covered in the refrigerator until ready to use.

Variation

Roasted Eggplant Spread

FULL DIET

Substitute roasted eggplant for the cauliflower. Preheat the oven to 375°F (190°C), cut 1 large eggplant in half lengthwise, poke skin side with a fork, and place skin side up on a baking sheet. Roast on the center oven rack for 40 minutes or until flesh is fully softened. Carefully scrape roasted eggplant flesh from skin, and allow flesh to cool completely. Proceed as directed.

Eggplant

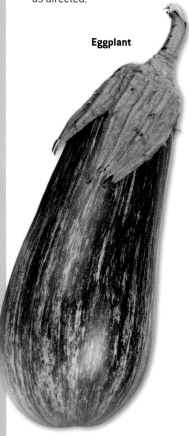

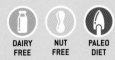

DAIRY FREE · **NUT FREE** · **PALEO DIET**

Garden Fresh Salsa

Toss together some sweet and ripe tomatoes, citrusy cilantro, a burst of lime acidity, a bit of optional chile pepper heat, and a dash of sea salt, and you have the makings of one of the simplest yet tastiest fresh salsas ever!

Prep Time
15 minutes

Makes
4 cups

Serving Size
$^1/_2$ cup

INGREDIENTS

3 cups seeded and chopped tomatoes
$^1/_2$ cup diced red onion
$^1/_2$ clove garlic, minced
$^1/_2$ tsp pure ground cumin
$^1/_2$ cup chopped fresh cilantro leaves
2 tbsp fresh lime juice
$^3/_4$ tsp sea salt
$^1/_4$ tsp ground black pepper
1 tbsp fresh green serrano, jalapeño, or poblano chiles, ribs and seeds removed (optional)

METHOD

1 In a food processor fitted with a metal chopping blade, pulse tomatoes, red onion, garlic, cumin, cilantro, lime juice, sea salt, black pepper, and chiles (if using) until ingredients are diced small and combined well.

2 Transfer to a bowl, cover tightly, and refrigerate until needed.

NUT FREE

Tzatziki Sauce

This cool and creamy, delectable dip is quick to make and lends a Greek flavor for dipping chips and vegetables or topping grilled meats and fish.

Makes
4 cups

Prep Time
15 minutes

Serving Size
$^1/_2$ cup

INGREDIENTS

2 cups homemade yogurt
2 cups peeled, seeded, and finely grated English cucumber
1 clove garlic, minced
1 tbsp lemon juice
2 tbsp fresh dill weed
1 tsp sea salt
$^1/_4$ tsp ground black pepper

METHOD

1 In a medium bowl, combine homemade yogurt, English cucumber, garlic, lemon juice, dill weed, sea salt, and black pepper.

2 Cover tightly, and refrigerate for 1 hour before serving.

NUT FREE **LOW FODMAP**

Parmesan Rosemary Tuiles

These thin, crisp crackers boast the fresh flavors of rosemary, lemon, and ground black pepper. You can vary the herbs and spices as you like.

Prep Time
10 minutes

Cook Time
5 minutes

Makes
12 tuiles

Serving Size
2 tuiles

INGREDIENTS

1 cup grated Parmigiano-Reggiano cheese
1 tbsp fresh rosemary
1 tsp lemon zest
1/2 tsp black pepper

METHOD

1 Preheat the oven to 400°F (200°C). Line a medium baking sheet with parchment paper.

2 In a small bowl, combine Parmigiano-Reggiano cheese, rosemary, lemon zest, and black pepper.

3 Place 1 heaping tablespoon cheese mixture onto the parchment paper, gently pressing down cheese to spread. Repeat 11 times, separating each cheese circle by 1 inch (2.5cm), for a total of 12 tuiles.

4 Bake on the middle oven rack for 5 minutes or until cheese is golden and crisp.

5 Cool completely, remove tuiles from the tray with a spatula, and rest on the curve of a round rolling pin until bent. Or lay them flat on a separate plate. If not serving immediately, store cooled tuiles tightly covered at room temperature for up to 1 week.

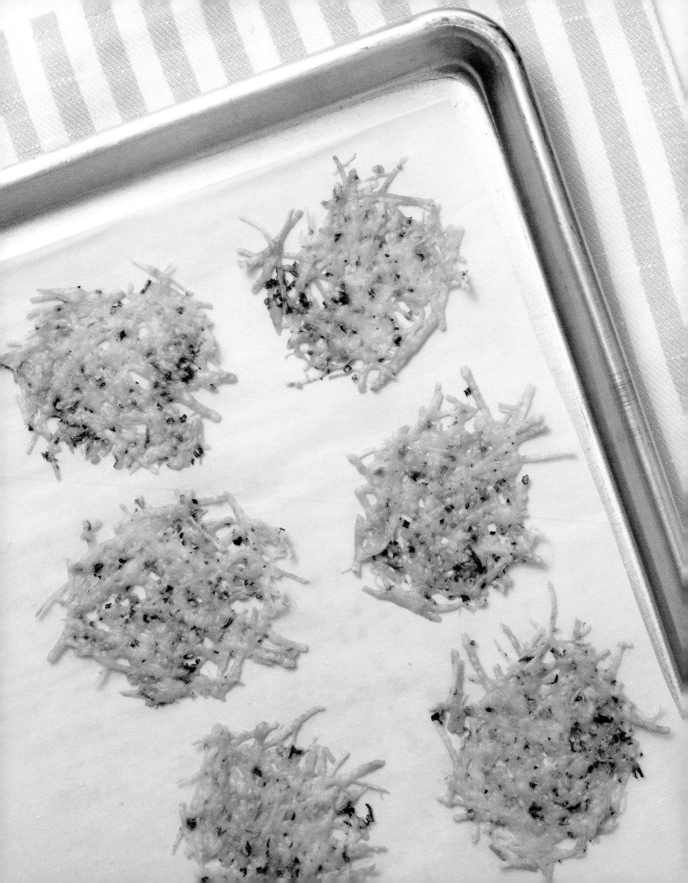

DAIRY FREE **PALEO DIET**

Three-Seed Crackers

When you want something crispy, crunchy, and salty, reach for these delightful crackers. They go great with chicken or tuna salad.

Prep Time
10 minutes

Cook Time
30 minutes

Makes
30 crackers

Serving Size
5 crackers

INGREDIENTS

1 cup hazelnut flour/meal

1 cup almond flour/meal

2 large pastured eggs

$1/4$ cup raw sunflower seeds, soaked and dried

$1/4$ cup raw pumpkin seeds, soaked and dried

$1/4$ cup raw sesame seeds, soaked and dried

1 tsp garlic powder

1 tsp onion powder

1 tsp sea salt

$1/4$ tsp black pepper

METHOD

1 Preheat the oven to 350°F (180°C).

2 In a food processor, chop hazelnut flour, almond flour, eggs, sunflower seeds, pumpkin seeds, sesame seeds, garlic powder, onion powder, sea salt, and black pepper until well combined and doughlike texture is reached.

3 Place dough on one side of a piece of parchment paper. Fold the parchment over on top of dough, and roll dough to a square with a consistent $1/8$ inch (3mm) thickness.

4 Using a dull knife, cut into 30 equal-size squares. Place on a baking sheet lined with parchment paper, and bake on the middle oven rack for 30 minutes or until lightly browned, using a spatula to turn halfway through.

Seeds add a nutritional boost by contributing helpful fatty acids, amino acids, zinc, selenium, and magnesium. If sunflower, pumpkin, and sesame aren't to your liking, you can substitute $1/4$ cup poppy seeds, $1/4$ cup hemp seeds, or $1/4$ cup flaxseeds.

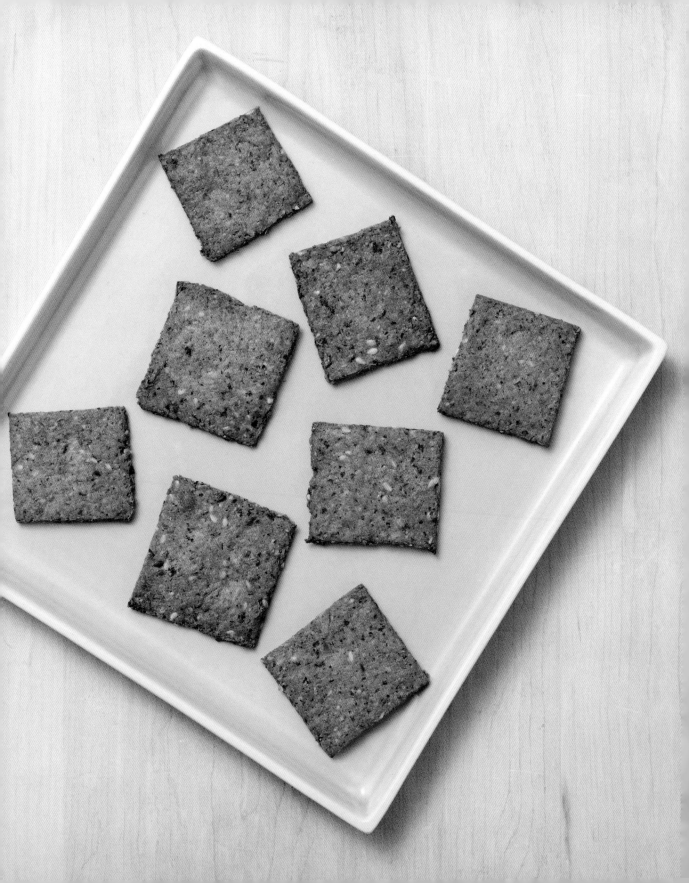

DAIRY FREE **PALEO DIET**

Nut Butter

When properly soaked, dried nuts are easy to turn into delicious nut butter. Far better than anything at your average grocery store, this nut butter is packed with healthy fat, protein, and energy.

Prep Time	Cook Time	Makes	Serving Size
5 minutes	10 minutes	4 cups	2 tablespoons

INGREDIENTS

4 cups soaked and dried nuts

4 tbsp coconut oil, melted

$\frac{1}{8}$ tsp sea salt

METHOD

1 In a food processor fitted with a metal chopping blade, pulse nuts until they resemble flour.

2 Add coconut oil and sea salt, and process, stopping to scrape down the sides of the food processor bowl as needed, until nut butter has reached your desired consistency.

3 Transfer nut butter to a glass jar, seal with the lid, and refrigerate for up to 6 months.

Variation

Coconut Butter

Pulse 4 cups unsweetened coconut flakes 10 times in a food processor fitted with a metal chopping blade and then process for 10 to 20 minutes, scraping down the sides of the food processor bowl as necessary. Store in a glass jar at room temperature for up to 6 months.

FULL DIET

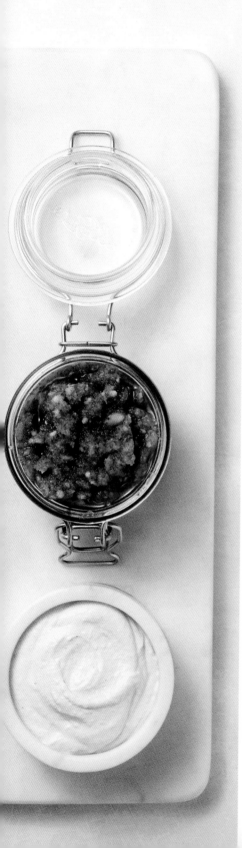

DAIRY FREE   **PALEO DIET**

Nut Cheese

If you have a dairy allergy, nut cheese, which can be spreadable or hard, can be a way to replace that cheesy goodness you miss. Take care, because nuts can sometimes be difficult to digest, even when properly prepared.

Prep Time
15 minutes

Makes
about 1 cup

Serving Size
3 tablespoons

INGREDIENTS

1 cup cashews or almonds, soaked overnight with 1 tsp sea salt, and skins removed (if needed)

3/4 cup water

2 tbsp coconut oil, melted

3 tsp lemon juice

1 clove garlic

1/8 tsp sea salt

METHOD

1 In a blender, process cashews, water, coconut oil, lemon juice, garlic, and sea salt for 5 to 7 minutes or until smooth.

2 Transfer mixture to a nut milk bag or a colander lined with cheesecloth, press down on solids or squeeze to remove excess liquid, and form cheese into a ball.

3 For a cremier cheese, serve immediately. For a harder cheese, refrigerate for 24 hours before serving.

DAIRY FREE **PALEO DIET**

Spiced Carrot Cake

Warm and fragrant spices, naturally sweet carrots, plump raisins, nutty walnuts, and a super-moist texture combine in this delightful cake.

Prep Time	Cook Time	Makes	Serving Size
15 minutes	45 minutes	1 cake; 16 pieces	1 piece

INGREDIENTS

$^1/_2$ cup raw honey

$^1/_2$ cup coconut oil, softened

5 large pastured eggs

2 tsp. organic pure vanilla extract

$3^1/_2$ cups almond flour

1 tsp pure ground ginger

3 tsp pure ground cinnamon

$^1/_2$ tsp pure ground nutmeg

$1^1/_2$ tsp baking soda

$^1/_2$ tsp sea salt

1 packed cup peeled and finely grated carrots

$^3/_4$ cup raw, unsalted walnuts, soaked and dried, and chopped

$^3/_4$ cup unsweetened, unsulfured raisins

METHOD

1 Preheat the oven to 325°F (170°C). Grease an 8×8-inch (20×20cm) glass baking dish with 1 teaspoon coconut oil.

2 With a mixer on medium, cream together honey and coconut oil. Add eggs one at a time, and beat until well combined. Add vanilla extract, and mix until combined.

3 In a separate bowl, combine almond flour, ginger, cinnamon, nutmeg, baking soda, and sea salt.

4 With the mixer on low, gradually add dry ingredients to wet ingredients and mix until well combined. Add carrots, walnuts, and raisins, and combine.

5 Pour into the baking dish, and bake on the middle oven rack for 45 minutes.

Variation

Zucchini Sunflower Cake with Currants

Substitute 1 cup grated zucchini for the carrots; $^3/_4$ cup raw, unsalted sunflower seeds for the walnuts; and $^3/_4$ cup unsweetened, unsulfured dried currants for the raisins. Proceed as directed.

FULL DIET

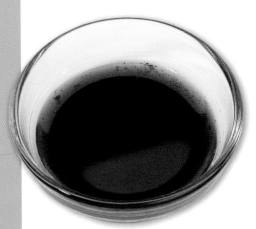

Organic pure vanilla extract

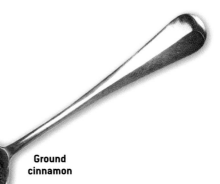

Ground cinnamon

DAIRY
FREE

PALEO
DIET

Hunger Buster Bars

Soft, chewy, and hearty, these balanced bites make a great snack between
meals or packed in school lunches. Make a double batch to last all week.

Prep Time	Cook Time	Makes	Serving Size
15 minutes	15 minutes	20 bars	1 bars

INGREDIENTS

¹/₂ cup raw whole almonds,
    soaked and dried

¹/₂ cup raw whole cashews,
    soaked and dried

¹/₂ cup raw pumpkin seeds,
    soaked and dried

¹/₂ cup raw whole peanuts,
    soaked and dried

2 cups unsweetened
    shredded coconut

¹/₂ cup raw sesame seeds,
    soaked and dried

¹/₂ cup raw sunflower
    seeds, soaked and dried

¹/₂ cup hemp seeds, soaked
    and dried

1 cup dried unsweetened,
    unsulfured figs

1¹/₂ cups homemade
    almond butter

³/₄ cup raw honey

1 tsp organic pure vanilla
    extract

METHOD

1 Preheat the oven to 350°F (180°C). Grease a 9×13-inch (23×33cm)
  rimmed baking sheet with 1 teaspoon coconut oil.

2 In a food processor fitted with a metal chopping blade, briefly pulse
  almonds, cashews, pumpkin seeds, and peanuts until roughly
chopped. Transfer to a large bowl.

3 To the bowl, add coconut, sesame seeds, sunflower seeds, hemp
  seeds, and figs, and mix to combine.

4 In a small saucepan over medium heat, melt almond butter and
  honey, whisking regularly, for 3 minutes. Remove from heat, add
vanilla extract, and stir to combine.

5 Pour almond butter mixture over nut, seed, and coconut mixture,
  and stir by hand to combine.

6 Using wet hands, spread mixture in an even layer on the prepared
  baking sheet, patting it down into a 1-inch (2.5cm) thick rectangle.
Bake on the middle oven rack for 15 minutes. Cool completely before
cutting. Store extras in a cool, dry place tightly covered for up to 1 week.

These bars are a breeze to customize. Instead of
the almond butter, try peanut butter, tahini
paste, cashew butter, or sunflower butter. In
place of the figs, you could use raisins, dried
apples, currants, apricots, or peaches. Feeling
spicy? Add ground cinnamon or ginger.

DAIRY FREE   **NUT FREE**   **PALEO DIET**

Very Berry "Ice Cream"

Cold, creamy, and delicate, this nutritionally enhanced version of the classic frozen dessert is incredibly rich and delightful.

Prep Time
15 minutes + 2 hours

Makes
4 cups

Serving Size
1/2 cup

INGREDIENTS

2 medium ripe bananas, peeled, cut into thin rounds, and frozen overnight

2 cups fresh or frozen strawberries, blueberries, raspberries, and/or blackberries (frozen overnight if fresh)

1 tbsp raw honey

METHOD

1 In a food processor fitted with a metal chopping blade, pulse frozen bananas and berries, stopping to scrape down the sides of the food processor bowl as needed, until a creamy texture is reached.

2 Add honey, and process to combine.

3 Transfer ice cream to an airtight container, cover, and freeze 2 hours or until frozen.

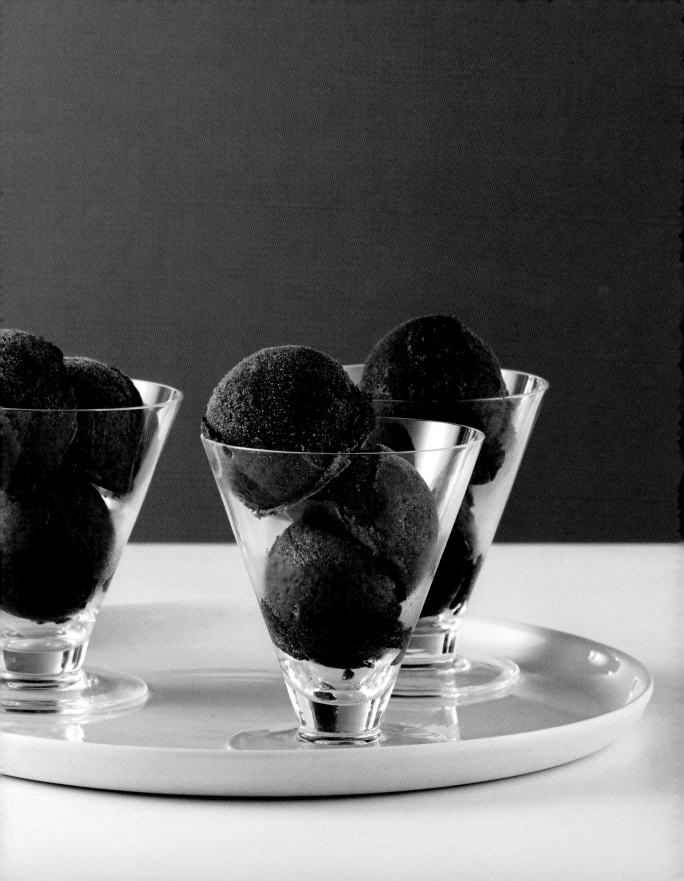

DAIRY FREE   PALEO DIET

Lemon Almond Flour Biscotti

These crunchy twice-baked bites of semisweet goodness have a nice hint of lemon and the nuttiness of whole chopped almonds.

Prep Time
10 minutes

Cook Time
40 minutes

Makes
40 biscotti

Serving Size
2 biscotti

INGREDIENTS

2 large eggs
1/4 cup raw honey
1/4 cup coconut oil
2 tbsp lemon zest
2 tbsp lemon juice
3 cups almond flour
1 cup hazelnut flour
1/2 cup flaxseed meal
1/2 cup chopped slivered almonds
1 tsp sea salt
2 tsp baking soda
1 1/2 tsp ground cinnamon

METHOD

1 Preheat the oven to 325°F (170°C). Line an 18×13-inch (46×33cm) baking sheet with parchment paper.

2 In a medium bowl, whisk together eggs, honey, coconut oil, lemon zest, and lemon juice.

3 In another medium bowl, combine almond flour, hazelnut flour, flaxseed meal, slivered almonds, sea salt, baking soda, and cinnamon. Fold wet ingredients into dry ingredients until well combined.

4 Place biscotti dough on a piece of parchment paper, and form into a log 1 1/2 inches (3.75cm) tall, 1 1/2 inches (3.75cm) wide, and 15 1/2 inches (39cm) long.

5 Bake on the middle oven rack for 20 minutes or until top is just browning. Allow to rest for 5 minutes before cutting. If log has started to crack on top, carefully squeeze to re-form.

6 Using a sharp chef's knife or serrated knife, cut log into 1/2-inch (1.25cm) cross-sectional pieces. Place cut pieces flat in a single layer on the parchment paper, and bake for 20 more minutes, turning biscotti halfway through the cook time. Cool completely before serving.

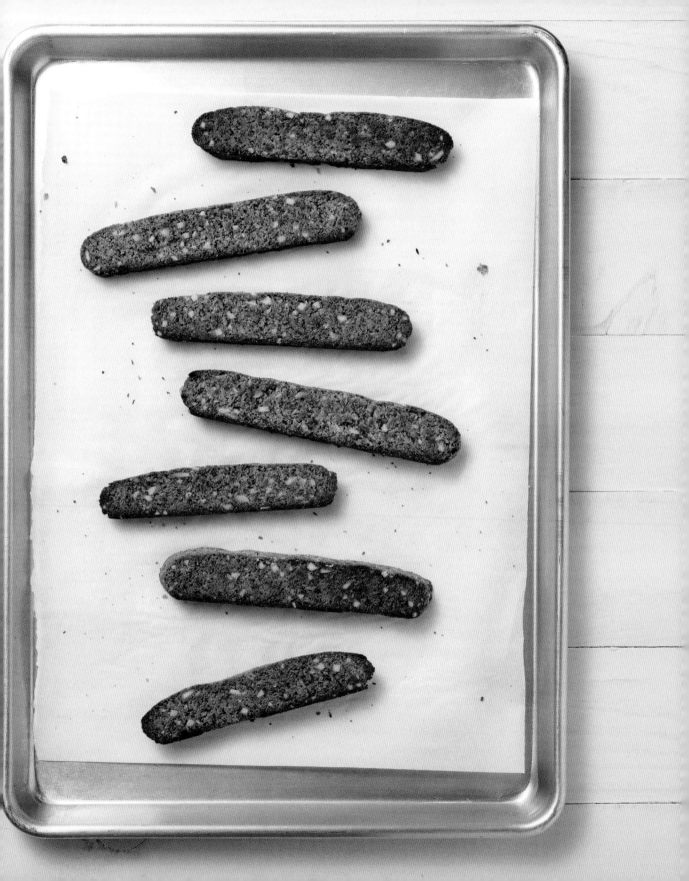

Index of Recipes by Type

**PALEO
DIET**

Index

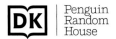

Publisher Mike Sanders
Acquisitions Editor Lori Cates Hand
Art & Design Director William Thomas
Cover Designer William Thomas
Book Designer Mandy Earey
Photographer Christopher Simpson
Food Stylist Laura Kinsey Dolph
Compositor Ayanna Lacey
Proofreader Cassie Armstrong
Indexer Heather McNeill

First American Edition, 2024
Published in the United States by DK Publishing
1745 Broadway, 20th Floor, New York, NY 10019

The authorized representative in the EEA is Dorling Kindersley
Verlag GmbH. Arnulfstr. 124, 80636 Munich, Germany

Library of Congress Catalog Number: 2023943368
ISBN: 978-0-7440-9250-9

DK books are available at special discounts when purchased
in bulk for sales promotions, premiums, fund-raising, or
educational use. For details, contact SpecialSales@dk.com

Printed and bound in China

www.dk.com

Reprinted from *Healthy Gut Cookbook*

ABOUT THE AUTHOR

Maya Gangadharan, FNTP, is a certified nutritional therapy
practitioner concentrating on gut health. She has a clinical
practice in Detroit. Visit intrinsicorigin.com to learn more.

ACKNOWLEDGMENTS

I would like to sincerely thank Gavin Pritchard and the team at DK
for all their work, guidance, and support. Extra thanks to Magda
Pecsenye for making the introduction. Much love and thanks to
my mother, Mary, who taught me all about healthy, home-
cooked meals, and to Rev, who always believes in me. Finally, to
my amazing NTA instructors Caroline Barringer, Janelle Johnson
Grove, and Christie Banners, and all my Ann Arbor 2015 NTP
classmates and group leaders—thanks for having my back and
teaching me so much. We've got this! —Maya

Special thanks to Gavin Pritchard, RDN, CSSD, CD-N, CDE, for
developing the recipes for the previous edition of this book;
Courtney Rinehold, RDN, CDN, CLT, and her clients for testing the
recipes; and Dana Angelo White for reviewing the recipes for this
edition.

PHOTO CREDITS

All images © Dorling Kindersley

10 Zygote Media Group, 12 Kristan Raines, 13 John Freeman, 18
Ruth Jenkinson, 21 Andy Crawford, 22 Dave King, 23 David Murray,
Ian O'Leary, William Reavell, Dave King, Ian O'Leary, 42 Roger
Dixon, David Murray, 38 Andy Crawford, 43 John Freeman, 46
Stuart West, 46 Lorenzo Vecchia, 47 Dave King, Chris Villano, 59
Stuart West, 62–63 Ali Donzé, 66 Dave King, 67 Steve Shott, 71
Lorenzo Vecchia, 72–73 Ali Donzé, 75 Dave King, 84 Will Heap, 85
William Reavell, 88 Dave King, 89 Steve Gorton, 92 Will Heap, 93
Dave King, 96 Dave King, 97 Will Heap, 99 Roger Phillips, 100 Andy
Crawford, 106 David Murray, 107 Clive Streeter, 110 Dave King,
111 William Reavell, 114 Ian O'Leary, 115 Steve Gorton, 117 Philip
Wilkins, 120 Claire Cordier, 124 David Murray and Jules Selmes,
125 Dave King, 130 David Murray, 131 Roger Dixon, 134 William
Reavell, 135 Ian O'Leary, 139 Geoff Dann, 143 Andy Crawford, 146
Steve Gorton, 149 Roger Dixon, 150 Will Heap, 151 Roger Dixon,
155 Roger Dixon, 159 Peter Anderson, 162 Roger Dixon, 163 William
Reavell, 165 Dave King, 167 Chris Villano, 168 Steve Gorton, 172
Lorenzo Vecchia, 176 Andy Crawford, 177 Roger Dixon, 180 Gary
Ombler, 181 William Reavell, 184 Dave King, 185 Roger Dixon, 190
Gary Ombler, 194 Will Heap, 199 Roger Dixon, 202 Lorenzo Vecchia,
210 William Reavel, Roger Dixon. Divider pages: Dave King, Roger
Dixon, Tim Ridley, Lorenzo Vecchia, Steve Gorton.